Safe Laparoscopic Cholecystectomy

Safe Laparoscopic Cholecystectomy

An Illustrated Atlas

Mohammad Ibrarullah MS, MCh
Professor and Senior Consultant
Department of Surgical Gastroenterology
Apollo Hospitals
Bhubaneswar, India

Sadiq S. Sikora MS (AIIMS), FACS, FRCS (Glas)
Director, Surgical Division
Institute of Digestive and HPB Sciences
Sakra World Hospital
Bangalore, India

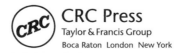

CRC Press
Taylor & Francis Group
Boca Raton London New York

CRC Press is an imprint of the
Taylor & Francis Group, an **informa** business

First edition published 2022
by CRC Press
6000 Broken Sound Parkway NW, Suite 300, Boca Raton, FL 33487-2742

and by Taylor & Francis Group
2 Park Square, Milton Park, Abingdon, Oxon, OX14 4RN

CRC Press is an imprint of Taylor & Francis Group, LLC

ISBN: 978-1-032-00521-8 (hbk)
ISBN: 978-1-032-00520-1 (pbk)
ISBN: 978-1-003-17454-7 (ebk)

DOI: 10.1201/9781003174547

Typeset in Minion
by SPi Technologies India Pvt Ltd (Straive)

Contents

Videos

The following supplemental videos are available at www.routledge.com/9781032005201.

Video	Title	Chapter
1.	Critical View of Safety	Chapter 4
2.	Critical View of Safety	Chapter 4*
3.	CVS in presence of low (anterior) cystic artery	Chapter 4
4.	CVS in presence of low (posterior) cystic artery	Chapter 4
5.	Cystic artery-superficial and deep division	Chapter 5
6.	Right hepatic artery hump	Chapter 5
7.	Cystic duct injury	Chapter 6*
8.	Cholecystohepatic duct	Chapter 7
9.	Fundus-first cholecystectomy	Chapter 8
10.	Subtotal cholecystectomy	Chapter 8*
11.	Acute gangrenous cholecystitis	Chapter 9
12.	Acute cholecystitis: Cystic duct stump management	Chapter 9*
13	Stone impacted in retrocholedochal cystic duct	Chapter 10
14.	Aberrant hepatic artery	Chapter 10
15.	Cholecysto-duodenal fistula	Chapter 10
16.	Completion cholecystectomy	Chapter 10*
17.	Cholecystectomy in EHPVO	Chapter 11
18.	Situs inversus	Chapter 12
19.	True left sided gallbladder	Chapter 12
20.	Management of bleeding during cholecystectomy	Chapter 14
21.	Biliovascular injury near miss	Chapter 15

*Not cited in the text

Foreword by Keith D. Lillemoe

Cholecystectomy remains the most common abdominal operation performed in the world. Whether the operation is performed, as in most cases as in 2021, laparoscopically or as an open procedure due to clinical indications, or even with the advent of new techniques such as robotic cholecystectomy, injury to the bile duct remains the most serious complication of the procedure. Although bile duct injuries have been observed with increased frequency since the original widespread use of the laparoscopic cholecystectomy in approximately 1990, it has only been in the last five years, primarily with the leadership of the Society of American Gastrointestinal and Endoscopic Surgeons (SAGES), who has made "safe cholecystectomy" the mission of their organization, that the prevention of bile duct injuries has been a major focus. This multi-pronged effort has focused on all aspects of the procedure and led to the recent publication of a landmark consensus conference published in 2020 by the Prevention of Bile Duct Injury Consensus Working Group.

Now this textbook, beautifully edited by Drs. Ibrarullah and Sikora, has provided an extensive review of this important topic, including preoperative evaluation to help with decision-making before the operating room, delineation of the relative anatomy and the steps of cholecystectomy, including establishing the critical view of safety.

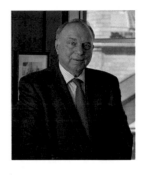

The management of the various aspects of the surgical procedure in both routine and special circumstances, such as acute cholecystitis, abnormal anatomy and other variants related to individual patients, is discussed. In addition, the authors have provided key information related to both troubleshooting problems during laparoscopic cholecystectomy and how to deal with errors and "near misses" in the operating room.

As this operation is of such primary importance to surgeons across the world, I believe this Atlas will be a valuable addition to the library of any general surgeon, any surgical training programme, or a busy clinical practice group in any country in the world. I congratulate the authors for their excellent work.

Keith D. Lillemoe, MD
Surgeon-in-Chief
Chief of Surgery
Massachusetts General Hospital
W. Gerald Austen Professor of Surgery
Harvard Medical School

Foreword by Raj Prasad

Excellence is a continuous process and not an accident

APJ Abdul Kalam
Former President of India

Laparoscopic cholecystectomy is the most common elective abdominal operation performed in healthcare systems across the world. Bile duct injuries of varying severity continue to occur, despite the procedure having been established for more than a quarter of a century. Almost all of them need some form of intervention, including biliary reconstructive surgery; the most severe needed extreme solutions like life-saving liver transplantations, a significant impact on quality of life, usage of additional health care resources and, in a small minority of cases, an unfortunate loss of life. Bile duct injury is a common cause for medico-legal suits filed against healthcare providers, including surgeons.

There is a wide variation in the performance and practice of this common operative procedure. It is performed by trainees to most experienced surgeons, with varied training backgrounds, general to specialist surgeons using multitude of technologies in terms of camera systems, telescopes and monitors. With all these variables, only knowledge and appropriate training provides a beacon for guidance towards excellence. Knowledge of variations in anatomy and pathology and training to recognize these variations and learning techniques to circumvent problems and avoiding common traps, recognizing when problems happen and seeking help are all key components of this continuous quest for safety.

And talking of beacons, the Surgical Gastroenterology department at Sanjay Gandhi

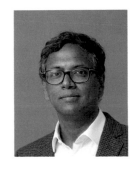

Postgraduate Institute of Medical Sciences (SGPGIMS), Lucknow, India springs to my mind. This department has had a unique impact on the surgical management of various abdominal diseases in India through its faculty and alumni. A generation of trainees benefited from the wisdom of this programme. How gallbladder disease is managed, from stones to cancer, and dealing with complications arising from managing the clinical problems has been a key area of interest for this department from the very beginning. Evidence-based medicine, improving safety and outcomes, teaching and training to the highest level have been among the important achievements of this extraordinary department and its illustrious faculty. It is of no surprise that two of its foremost alumni have joined hands to produce this well-resourced treasure trove of an atlas.

The chapters and list of videos make essential reading and viewing for anyone intending to eliminate risks from cholecystectomy. Despite being part of the laparoscopic cholecystectomy journey since 1992, I've gained fresh insights into anatomy, pathology and techniques. The formatting of chapters lends itself for easy reading and effective learning. Much-needed emphasis has been placed on the 'Critical View of Safety'. The importance of Rouviere's sulcus and its variations are well depicted. The quality of images, I have to say, is exceptional. Whilst it is difficult to pick out my favourites, I enjoyed very much the chapters on anatomy, acute cholecystitis, cirrhosis and portal hypertension and completion cholecystectomy. The chapter on 'near misses' is an invaluable collection of cases that provide insights into how problems can happen easily if principles were abandoned. It highlights the essential steps that cannot be circumvented in the practice of safe cholecystectomy. I congratulate Sadiq and Ibrar, and their collaborators, for this excellent addition to the library of biliary and general surgeons and also surgical trainees.

I have no doubt that this huge effort, in the years to come, will not only fulfil the aspirations of Sadiq and Ibrar as a road map for safe cholecystectomy, but also contribute to the growing legacy of a great department of surgical gastroenterology.

Raj Prasad, MS, MCh, FRCS
Consultant Surgeon
Hepatobiliary and Transplant Unit
Leeds Teaching Hospitals
Leeds, UK

Conflict of interest – I was fortunate to be guided by the knowledge, wisdom and experience of these two exceptional surgeons during my formative years in Lucknow and have reaped the benefits ever since.

Preface

Gallstone disease is highly prevalent across the world, with rates varying from 20% in the USA, 9–21% in Europe and 10% in Japan. In India, the prevalence rates are higher in North India, with rates varying from 6 to 13%. Cholecystectomy is the commonest abdominal operation performed across the world, with around 300,000 cholecystectomies performed yearly in the USA. Bile duct injury (BDI) is a dreaded complication of cholecystectomy. Notwithstanding the low incidence of BDI, the burden of this complication is considered very high due to the large number of patients undergoing cholecystectomy across the globe.

The conduct of cholecystectomy has also undergone a paradigm shift in the last two decades. Open cholecystectomy was the standard of care and the authors are privy to the evolution and journey of cholecystectomy in India. An open cholecystectomy with a subhepatic drain and a five-day hospital stay was the norm in the early 1980s until the laparoscopic revolution which was ushered in and adopted as standard of care after the National Institutes of Health (NIH) consensus in 1992.

During our stint at the Sanjay Gandhi Postgraduate Institute of Medical Sciences (SGPGIMS), a tertiary referral institute in North India, we not only managed a large number of patients referred with bile duct injuries but also experienced the medical, social and financial implications associated with this complication. Gallstones being highly prevalent, cholecystectomy is being performed in many small hospitals with limited facilities and by inadequately trained surgeons. Added to this is the high variability and uncertainties of the anatomy and pathology of the biliary system. Moreover, laparoscopic cholecystectomy was adopted in clinical practice without proper training and credentialing, especially in the initial wave. It is therefore imperative that the training of young surgeons is taken seriously to ensure a culture and practice of cholecystectomy that is safe *sans* any major complications.

There is a common quote made in relation to laparoscopic cholecystectomy– 'there are two categories of surgeons – one who has cut the bile duct and one who will cut the bile duct'. Based on our experience we would like to change this to 'a cholecystectomy is not just a gallbladder removed but a Bile Duct saved'. We concur with Keith Lillemoe who said – 'Surgery is not a mindless "rock, paper, scissors" game where outcome is determined by chance. Surgeons must take responsibility for the safe conduct of the procedure and the consequences of their own errors'.

The atlas provides an illustrative (including selected videos) step-wise guide for cholecystectomy, documents the variations of biliary and vascular anatomy relevant to cholecystectomy, summarizes the key concepts and highlights important considerations and techniques in difficult situations. The authors went through hours of video recordings of the procedures, selected and edited each frame of the images and videos which were important, relevant and that addressed critical issues. The project of the *Atlas of Safe Cholecystectomy* was driven by two objectives: firstly, to document and share the vagaries and complexities of a common operation; and secondly, to provide a resource for students, trainee and practicing surgeons to understand key concepts in performing a safe cholecystectomy in simple and complicated situations.

Safe cholecystectomy is a *passion and mission* for us. We have conducted several single-theme training courses on 'Safe Cholecystectomy' in various parts of India in our drive to fulfil this mission. The author (SSS) has been a member of the SELSI Expert Working Group and the International Multisociety Prevention of Bile Duct Injury Consensus Working Group that has developed consensus guidelines in the practice of safe cholecystectomy.

We hope this Atlas fulfils the objectives that we envisaged and provides a meaningful resource for the young surgeons to navigate the complexities encountered in the management of gallstone disease.

Acknowledgements

We sincerely thank our team members for their active participation in our endeavour to propagate the concept and practice of 'Safe Cholecystectomy'.

Team, Apollo Hospitals, Bhubaneswar

- Dr Sadananda Meher
- Dr MS Modi
- Dr Hamza Wani
- Dr Uppalapati Srinivasulu
- Dr Laxminarayan Mohanty
- Dr Ambika P Dash
- Dr Salil Parida
- Dr Pramod K Samantray
- Prakash Ch Panda
- Satish Ch Satpathy
- Nirakara Mohanty

Team, Sakra World Hospital, Bangalore
- Dr Somyaa Khuller
- Dr Gayatri Balachandran

- Dr Manoj Kumar
- Dr Kishore GSB
- Mr Girish
- Mr Chembian

Our special thanks to:

- Dr Sadananda Meher, Consultant, Minimally Invasive Surgery, Apollo Hospitals, Bhubaneswar, for his meticulous technique and documentation of some of the most complex cases presented in this Atlas.
- Dr Rahul Mahadar, Consultant, Minimally Invasive and GI Surgery, Jeevanshree Hospital, Dombivli, Mumbai, for his contribution 'True left-sided gallbladder'.
- Dr Manoj Kumar Sahu, Professor and Head. Dept of Gastroenterology, IMS and SUM Hospital, Bhubaneswar for the EUS image.

The authors acknowledge Dr Somyaa Khuller and Dr Gayatri Balachandran, Sakra World Hospital, Bangalore, for their contribution in editing and annotating the videos. Their contribution has added a unique dimension to the Atlas.

Authors

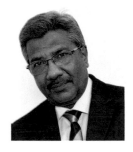

Dr Mohammad Ibrarullah is currently serving as Professor and Senior Consultant in the Department of Surgical Gastroenterology, Apollo Hospitals, Bhubaneswar, India. An alumnus from Sanjay Gandhi Postgraduate Institute of Medical Sciences, Lucknow, he has been associated with SV Institute of Medical Sciences, Tirupati and Sriramachandra Medical College, Chennai as Professor and Head of the Department of Surgical Gastroenterology in the past. He was awarded 'Travel Scholar' by the International Society of Surgery foundation, USA and Japan Surgical Society in 1995. He has more than 100 research publications and book chapters to his credit on HPB surgery and bile duct injury in particular and he has also authored the internationally acclaimed *Atlas of Diagnostic Endoscopy*, 3rd edition (CRC Press/Taylor & Francis, USA).

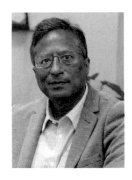

Dr Sadiq S. Sikora is currently the Director, Surgical Division, Institute of Digestive and HPB Sciences, Sakra World Hospital, Bangalore. He is an alumnus of AIIMS, New Delhi where he did his surgical training and senior residency. He was on the faculty of the prestigious SGPGIMS, Lucknow from 1991 to 2005. A Fellow of the American College of Surgeons and also of the Royal College of Surgeons (Glasgow), he is the recipient of several awards. He is credited with more than 125 research publications and has authored several chapters in national and international textbooks. His passion for 'Safe Cholecystectomy' is acknowledged globally. He was a member of the International Multisociety Working Group to formulate guidelines for Safe Cholecystectomy, and also a member of the Society of Endoscopic and Laparoscopic Surgeons of India (SELSI) Working Groups on compiling the 'SELSI Consensus Statement for Safe Cholecystectomy - Prevention and Management of Bile Duct injury'. He has conducted several dedicated courses for 'Safe Cholecystectomy' across India. His primary area of interest is in the management of post-cholecystectomy bile duct injuries to which he has contributed by way of lectures delivered at international and national conferences and has contributed several research articles on this subject.

Abbreviations

AA	Aberrant artery	GDA	Gastroduodenal artery
ASA	American Society of	HA	Hepatic artery
	Anaesthesiologist's	HC triangle	Hepatocystic triangle
ACA	Accessary artery	HDL	Hepatoduodenal ligament
ANT	Anterior	HM pouch	Hartman's pouch
ASGE	American Society for	ICG	Indocyanine green
	Gastrointestinal Endoscopy	IOC	Intraoperative cholangiogram
CA	Cystic artery	LFT	Liver function test
CBD	Common bile duct	LHA	Left hepatic artery
CD	Cystic duct	LN	Lymph node (Cystic)
CDF	Cholecystoduodenal fistula	LUS	Laparoscopic ultrasound
CHA	Common hepatic artery	M	Mucosa
CHD	Common hepatic duct	MRCP	Magnetic resonance
CH duct	Cholecystohepatic duct		cholangio-pancreatogram
CRP	C-reactive protein	PDS	Polydioxanone
CP	Cystic plate	Post	Posterior
CT	Computerized tomography	RHA	Right hepatic artery
D	Duodenum	RPP	Right portal pedicle
DCA	Deep branch of cystic artery	SCA	Superficial branch of cystic artery
FC	Fluorescent cholangiography	Seg 4	Segment 4
FL	Falciform ligament	SVD	Subvesicle duct
GB	Gallbladder	UF	Umbilical fissure
GBM	Gallbladder mesentery	USG	Ultrasonography

Introduction

Laparoscopic cholecystectomy (LC) is the commonest abdominal surgery performed across the globe. In the majority of cases, the surgery is uneventful and can be performed as a day care procedure. The incidence of biliary complications following LC is in the range 0.36–1.5%. The actual figure, however, could still be higher and assumes significance because of the huge number of cholecystectomies performed around the world. Bile duct injury (BDI), the most sinister of all the complications of LC, can be a cause for prolonged morbidity, increased hospitalization cost and possible litigation. Though lack of experience, anatomical variations and inflammatory alteration of anatomy are considered the underlying factors, in more than 90% of cases the injury can be directly attributed to 'perception error'. Two of the most common perception errors that can have serious consequences are mistaking the common bile duct for a cystic duct and misidentifying the right hepatic artery as cystic artery. The entire concept of safe cholecystectomy focuses on dealing with these two structures during surgery.

Extrahepatic bilio-vascular anatomy is complex and extremely variable. Anatomical variations have been recorded in nearly half of the patients undergoing laparoscopic cholecystectomy. Though not all of the variations are clinically significant, those occurring in the vicinity of the gallbladder must be identified in order to prevent complications during cholecystectomy.

The infundibular approach for cholecystectomy is still the most common technique practiced by many surgeons. In this approach, the surgeon dissects the infundibulum of the gallbladder, encircles the ductal structure and adjacent blood vessel, presuming these to be cystic duct and artery respectively, applies clips and divides.

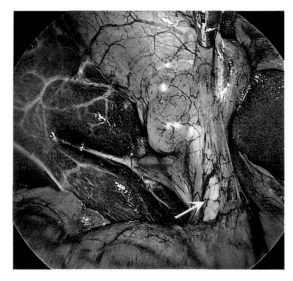

Figure 1.1 Perception error. Common bile duct (arrow) appears as cystic duct.

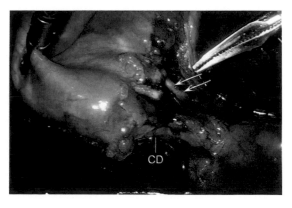

Figure 1.2 RHA (arrows) masquerading as cystic artery (*refer to Chapter 5 for details*).

DOI: 10.1201/9781003174547-1

In this scenario, not dissecting the hepatocystic triangle and defining the structures clearly, may lead to mistakenly perceiving the common bile duct as the cystic duct (Fig 1.1) and the right hepatic artery (normal/aberrant) as the cystic artery (Fig 1.2), thereby causing injury.

The concept of 'Critical View of Safety' (CVS) was first introduced by Strasberg in 1995. This envisages the clear identification of the cystic duct and artery before these are clipped and divided. The three components of CVS are: *clearing the hepatocystic triangle of all fibro-fatty tissue; dissecting distal one-third of the gallbladder off the cystic plate; and identification of only two structures, i.e., cystic duct and artery entering the gallbladder.* In about 90–95% of patients it is possible to establish CVS, identify the structures clearly and then divide, ensuring that the cholecystectomy is performed safely. On the other hand, recent surveys have indicated that in almost all cases of bile duct injury the surgeon did not establish CVS prior to dividing the 'cystic duct'.

The present book addresses these and several other issues in the context of 'Safe Cholecystectomy'. The procedure has been broken down into individual components and each aspect is demonstrated with detailed pictures from the procedure. The book is also supplemented with selected videos. This atlas attempts to enhance the understanding of the normal anatomy and the variations and approach to cholecystectomy in these situations for trainees and practicing surgeons.

2

Evaluation of Patients with Gallstone Disease

Patients with gallstones disease, as with any other patients, have to undergo a complete clinical evaluation for the disease-related issues and also general issues pertaining to fitness for surgery. The evaluation of these patients should proceed along two lines:

1. **General evaluation** – Assessment and optimization of comorbidities – pulmonary and cardiac status and control of diabetes. This is especially relevant in elderly patients with multiple comorbidities, where the status of the patient determines the approach to treatment of gallstone disease. Poor pulmonary function due to chronic obstructive pulmonary disease (COPD) and cardiac dysfunction have to be optimized.
2. **Disease evaluation** – Complete history and physical examination, blood counts, liver function test and renal function test are important. Liver function derangements can be seen in patients with acute cholecystitis, common bile duct stones or associated pancreatitis.
   a. USG (Fig 2.1) is the primary investigation for diagnosis and determination of complications related to gallstone disease. The following information should be sought on the USG.

    i. Gallbladder – distended or contracted
    ii. Number, size and position of the gallstone/s
    iii. Gallbladder wall thickness – focal, diffuse, mass formation; pericholecystic oedema/fluid
    iv. Sonographic Murphy's sign
    v. Liver – echotexture, enlargement
    vi. Status of intrahepatic bile duct, common hepatic duct and common bile duct – normal/dilated and presence of stone/s.
    vii. Pancreas – normal or enlarged; presence of any peripancreatic fluid suggestive of pancreatitis

  b. Contrast enhanced CT scan (Fig 2.2) is recommended in patients with acute cholecystitis, suspected complications like empyema, perforation or pancreatitis. CT scan is also recommended in patients having focal wall thickening (Fig 2.3) or mass lesion seen on USG.
  c. MRCP (Fig 2.4) and EUS – should be performed when there is suspicion of common bile duct stones (discussed later)

DOI: 10.1201/9781003174547-2

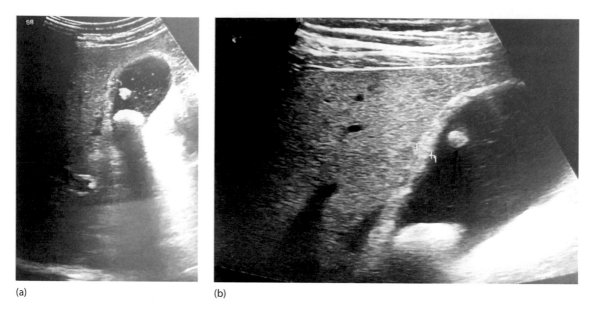

(a)　　　　　　　　　　　　(b)

Figure 2.1 Ultrasound image **(a, b)** Distended gallbladder, stone impacted at neck. A thin hypoechoic layer in the gallbladder wall is suggestive of wall oedema in a patient of acute cholecystitis.

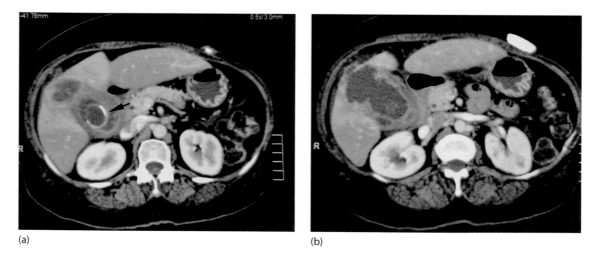

(a)　　　　　　　　　　　　(b)

Figure 2.2 Acute cholecystitis with gallbladder perforation. **(a, b)** Contrast enhanced CT scan of gallbladder showing grossly thickened gallbladder wall with perforation at the fundus. Note a large size stone(arrow) in the lumen exhibiting rim calcification.

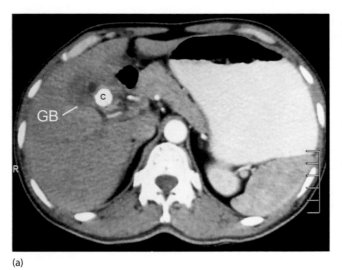

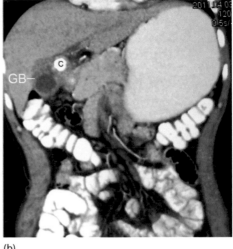

(a)   (b)

Figure 2.3 Xanthogranulomatous cholecystitis: **(a, b)** Contrast enhanced CT scan showing thickening of the gallbladder wall with near complete obliteration of the lumen. A large calcified stone with its nidus (appearing as 'C') is seen impacted at the neck. Gallbladder cancer was the preoperative diagnosis in this patient

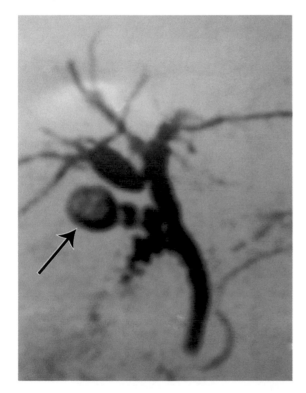

Figure 2.4 MRCP showing a stone in the gallbladder stump (arrow), in a patient who had previously undergone cholecystectomy. Long cystic duct is seen. CHD, CBD are normal with no stones. Low insertion of right posterior sectoral duct is visualised.

PREOPERATIVE EVALUATION FOR ANTICIPATED DIFFICULTIES DURING CHOLECYSTECTOMY

The first step towards conduct of safe cholecystectomy includes assessment for any intraoperative difficulty that may necessitate conversion to open cholecystectomy. During operative planning and intraoperative decision-making, the surgeon should consider the following factors that potentially increase the difficulty of laparoscopic cholecystectomy (Table 2.1).

Table 2.1 Factors associated with difficult laparoscopic cholecystectomy

Male sex	Enlarged liver
Old age	Liver cirrhosis
Obesity	Adhesions from
Anatomic variation/s	previous abdominal
Chronic cholecystitis	surgery
(thick-walled gallbladder)	Cancer of gallbladder
Cystic duct stone/s	and/or biliary tract,
Emergency	Bilio-digestive fistula
cholecystectomy	Limited surgical
	experience

Source: Brunt LM, Deziel DJ, Telem DA et al. Safe cholecystectomy multi-society practice guideline and state of the art consensus conference on prevention of bile duct injury during cholecystectomy. *Annals of Surgery* 2020; 272: 3–23.

A scoring system has been proposed that predicts conversion from laparoscopic to open cholecystectomy (Table 2.2).

Table 2.2 Conversion from Laparoscopic to Open Cholecystectomy (CLOC) risk score

Factors	Score
Age	
<30	0
30–39	2
40–69	3
70+	5
Gender	
Female	0
Male	1
Indication	
Colic/Pancreatitis	0
Acute cholecystitis	2
CBD Stone	3
ASA	
1	0
2	2
3	3
Gallbladder wall	
Normal	0
Thick walled	1
CBD diameter	
Normal	0
Dilated	1

Note: Score >6 identified patients at high risk of conversion.

Source: Sutcliffe RP, Hollyman M, Hodson J et al. Preoperative risk factors for conversion from laparoscopic to open cholecystectomy: a validated risk score derived from a prospective U.K. database of 8820 patients. *HPB* 2016; 18: 922–928.

PREDICTION AND DIAGNOSIS OF COMMON BILE DUCT STONE

Common bile duct stones are present in 5–20% of patients undergoing cholecystectomy. Asymptomatic CBD stones are present in <5% of patients with normal liver function test and USG findings. USG diagnoses CBD stones with a sensitivity of 71% and a specificity of 91% (Fig 2.5). MRCP (Figs 2.6 and 2.7) and EUS (Fig 2.8) are the two most reliable modalities to diagnose CBD stone with a sensitivity and specificity of more than 95% for each.

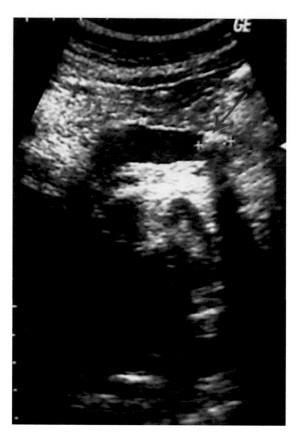

Figure 2.5 Dilated common bile duct with a stone at the lower end (arrow) on ultrasonography.

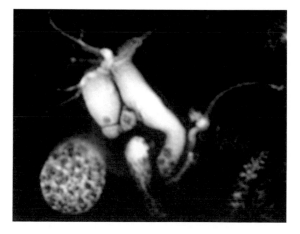

Figure 2.6 MRCP showing multiple small calculi in gallbladder and CBD.

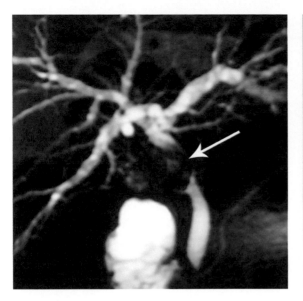

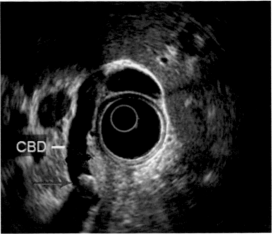

Figure 2.8 Endoscopic ultrasound showing dilated CBD and an impacted stone (arrow) with acoustic shadow at the lower end of bile duct.

Figure 2.7 A large calculus (arrow) is impacted in the mid-CBD in an eccentric manner. Dilatation of CBD proximal to the obstruction, a 'peg'-shaped deformity of the bile duct below the obstructing calculus is suggestive of Mirizzi's syndrome.

The American Society of Gastrointestinal Endoscopy (ASGE) in the practice guidelines identified predictors of CBD stones and stratified the patients into high, intermediate and low risk categories (Table 2.3). On the basis of that we propose an algorithm of management (Figure 2.9).

Table 2.3 Predictors of CBD stone/s and risk stratification

	Parameters	Risk Stratification
Very Strong Predictors	Cholangitis Preoperative jaundice (>4 mg%) USG evidence of CBD stone	**High Risk (>50%)** Any of very strong predictors or two of strong predictors
Strong Predictors	Dilated CBD on USG Jaundice (1.8–4 mg%)	**Intermediate Risk (10–50%)** All remaining patients
Moderate Predictors	Abnormal LFT other than bilirubin Pancreatitis (raised amylase) Age >55 years	**Low Risk (<10%)** None of the predictors are present

Source: ASGE Standards of Practice Committee. Maple JT, Ben-Menachem T, Anderson MA et al. The role of endoscopy in the evaluation of suspected choledocholithiasis. *Gastrointestinal Endoscopy* 2010; 7: 1–9.

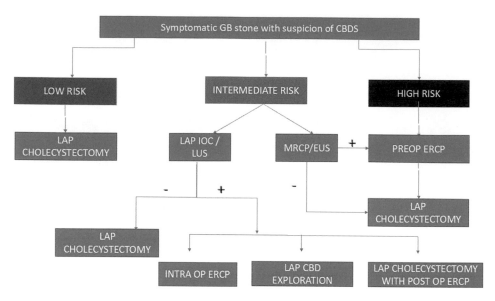

Figure 2.9 Approach to patients with suspected CBD stones according to the risk stratification. CBDS – common bile duct stone; (+) CBD stone present; (−) CBD stone absent.

3

Surgical Anatomy Relevant to Cholecystectomy

Biliary anatomy is extremely variable to the extent that *variation is a norm*. An adequate knowledge of extrahepatic bilio-vascular anatomy is paramount to the safe conduct of laparoscopic cholecystectomy. Though anatomical variations are noted in nearly half of the cases, all of it may not be appreciated during surgery. In this chapter, we have presented the anatomy, its variations and landmarks that the operating surgeon will encounter and has to be aware of while performing laparoscopic cholecystectomy. The relevant anatomy during cholecystectomy can be broadly described as follows.

Rule of Two!!

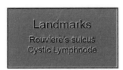
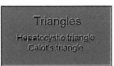
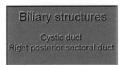
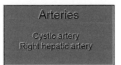

ROUVIERE'S SULCUS

Rouviere's sulcus (RS) is an important extrahepatic landmark in cholecystectomy. RS is visible inferior to the gallbladder in 70–90% of cases and represents the plane of the extrahepatic portal pedicle. Dissection during laparoscopic cholecystectomy should remain anterior/ventral to this plane. An imaginary line (R4U) that passes from the sulcus, across the base of segment IV to the umbilical fissure is an important guide for safe surgery (Fig 3.1). Dissection should commence above this line/plane to safeguard vital structures in the hepatoduodenal ligament. Several morphological types of RS have been proposed[1,2]. Based on our observation we also propose an addition to the described types (Table 3.1).

Table 3.1 Classification of Rouviere's sulcus (Figs 3.2–3.12)

Type		Incidence
Type 0	Absent or rudimentary sulcus	10–30%
Type 1 / Deep:	Deep sulcus with measurable dimensions	61–71%
1A / open:	*Medial end of the sulcus open, fused lateral end*	
1B / closed:	*Lateral end of the sulcus open, fused medial end*	
1C:	*Sulcus fused in the middle**	
Type 2 / Slit:	Shallow sulcus (the depth and width are barely measurable)	23–30%
Type 3 / Scar:	Completely fused, appearing as a white linear scar	6–8%
Type 4:	Double sulcus*	

Sources: Singh M, Prasad N. *Journal of Minimal Access Surgery.* 2017; 13: 89–95.
Lazarus L, Luckrajh JS, Kinoo S M, Singh B. *European Journal of Anatomy.* 2018; 22: 389–395.
* Based on our observation

DOI: 10.1201/9781003174547-3

The sulcus may lie transverse, oblique or rarely vertical. In 70% of cases, it contains the right posterior sectoral pedicle. Additionally, it may contain the vein to segment VI, anterior sectoral pedicle or the cystic vein in 25%, 5% and 18%, respectively

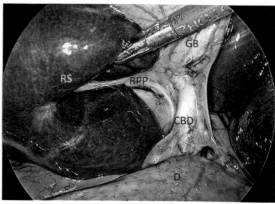

Figure 3.3 Type 1A - The transversely placed sulcus is continuous with hilum. The right portal pedicle and its constituents can be seen entering the sulcus.

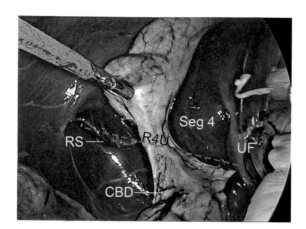

Figure 3.1 R4U line: An imaginary line (yellow dotted line) passing through Rouviere's sulcus, base of segment 4 and Umbilical fissure. Safe dissection for cholecystectomy should remain above this plane.

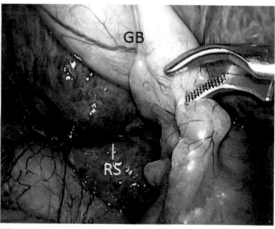

(a)

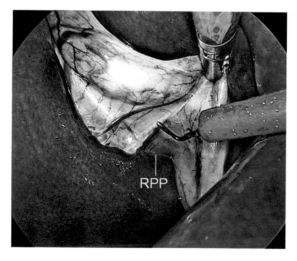

Figure 3.2 Type 0 - Absent Rouviere's sulcus.

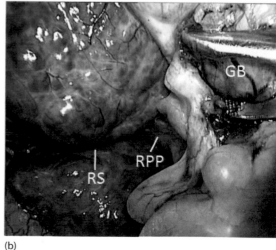

(b)

Figure 3.4 Type 1A **(a, b)**. Cirrhosis of liver with irregular hypertrophy of segments has resulted in an accentuated sulcus.

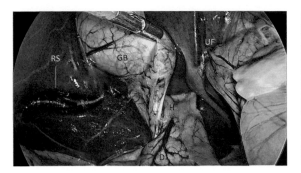

Figure 3.5 Type 1B - The sulcus is closed medially (towards hilum).

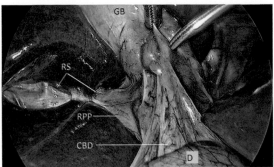

Figure 3.8 Type 1C - The right portal pedicle is clearly seen inside the sulcus

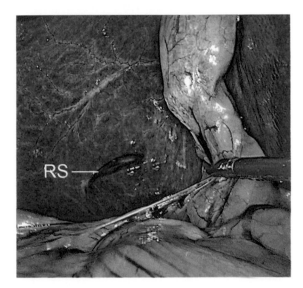

Figure 3.6 Type 1B - The sulcus is closed medially (towards hilum).

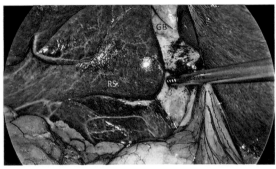

Figure 3.9 Type 2 - A slit like very shallow sulcus.

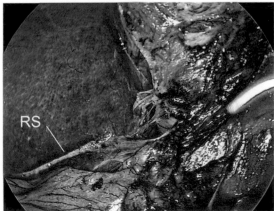

Figure 3.10 Type 2 - A slit like very shallow sulcus.

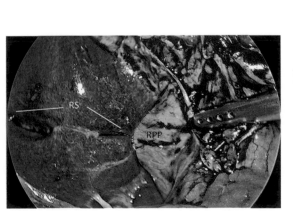

Figure 3.7 Type 1 C - The sulcus is fused in the middle.

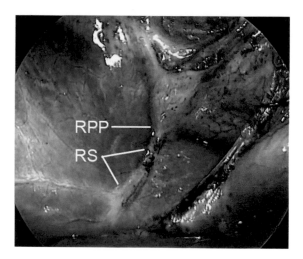

Figure 3.11 Type 3 - The sulcus is completely obliterated and appears like a scar.

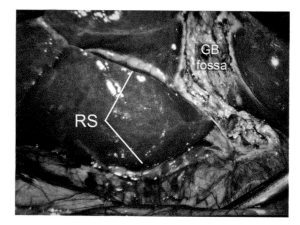

Figure 3.12 Type 4 – Double sulcus.

CYSTIC LYMPH NODE

Cystic lymph node is a constant landmark in the hepatocystic triangle and serves as a guide to the cystic artery (Figs 3.14–3.17). The artery runs in close proximity to the lymph node, usually behind and occasionally in front of the lymph node. It is a

safe practice to dissect the artery close to the node. The cystic line is an imaginary line running through the cystic lymph node and parallel to the hepatoduodenal ligament. Dissection lateral to this imaginary line marks the safe zone of dissection preventing injury to the RHA and the CHD/CBD. The intersection of the RU4 line and the cystic lymph node line defines the safe zone of dissection (Fig 3.13).

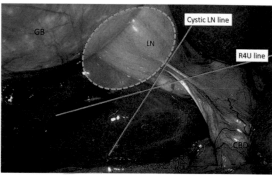

Figure 3.13 Cystic LN line, R4U line and the safe zone of dissection (dotted green circle).

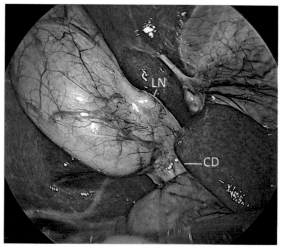

Figure 3.14 Typical location of cystic lymph node.

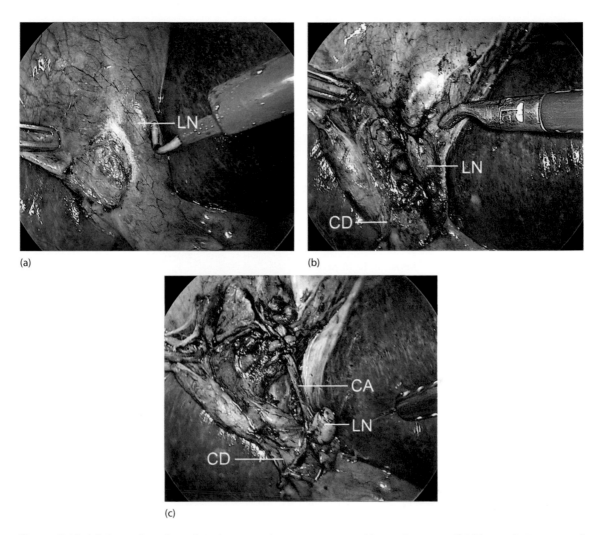

(a)   (b)

(c)

Figure 3.15 **(a)** Cystic lymph node in its normal position, covered by peritoneum. **(b)** The node is exposed as the overlying peritoneum is divided and dissection carried out. **(c)** The cystic artery lying behind the lymph node. Note the position of the lymph node after complete dissection of the hepatocystic triangle.

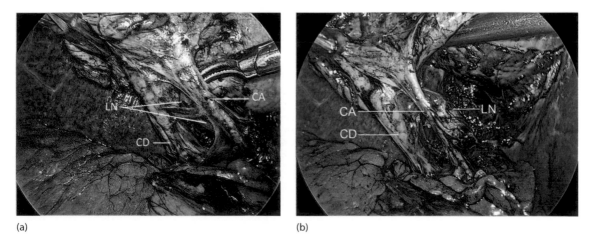

(a)   (b)

Figure 3.16 **(a)** Large cystic lymph node behind cystic artery. **(b)** The lymph node is adherent to the artery, seen after dissecting the hepatocystic triangle.

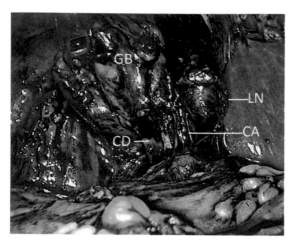

Figure 3.17 Enlarged cystic lymph node in acute cholecystitis in close proximity to cystic artery.

CYSTIC DUCT

The cystic duct is usually 2–4 cm long and 2–3 mm wide. It joins the common hepatic duct in different configurations (Figure 3.18). The most common variant is an angular insertion of CD in 75% (Fig 3.19), followed by a parallel CD in 20% (Figs 3.20 and 3.21) and a spiral CD in 5% (Figs 3.22 and 3.23) of cases. It may occasionally join the right hepatic duct or right sectoral duct in 0.6–2.3% of cases. It is rarely absent, but more often the absence is due to inflammatory shortening (Fig 3.24) or erosion by a stone, as in Mirizzi syndrome. *For a safe cholecystectomy, it is important to display its junction with gallbladder rather than the point of insertion into the CBD.*

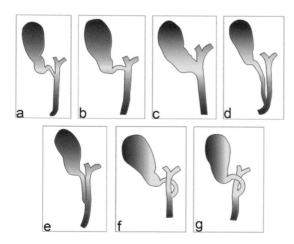

Figure 3.18 Cystic duct variants **(a)** angular insertion, **(b)** high insertion, **(c)** absent CD, **(d)** parallel CD, **(e)** parallel CD fused with the CBD, **(f)** spiral posterior CD, **(g)** spiral anterior CD.

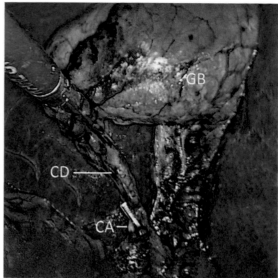

Figure 3.19 Normal insertion of the cystic duct (angular variety).

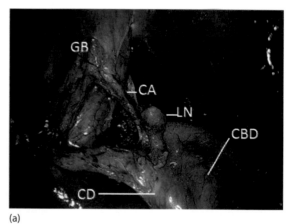

(a)

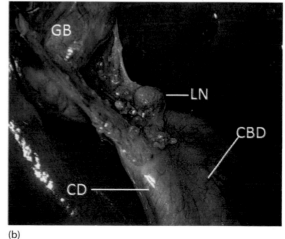

(b)

Figure 3.20 **(a, b)** Parallel cystic duct.

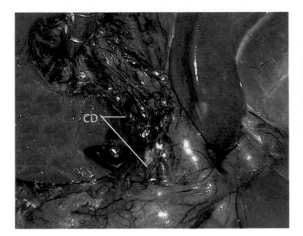

Figure 3.21 Parallel cystic duct.

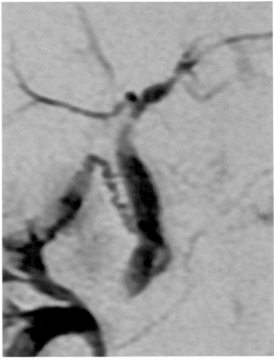

Figure 3.23 Spiral variety of cystic duct on MRCP.

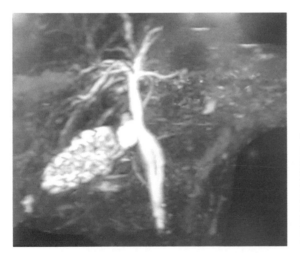

Figure 3.22 Spiral variety of cystic duct on MRCP.

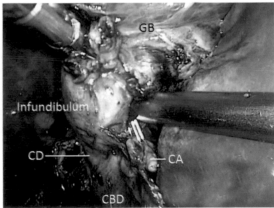

Figure 3.24 Absent cystic duct: Obliteration of the cystic duct resulting in the appearance of a sessile gallbladder. The interface between gallbladder and CBD can be appreciated as a groove demarcating the two structures.

SUBVESICLE DUCT

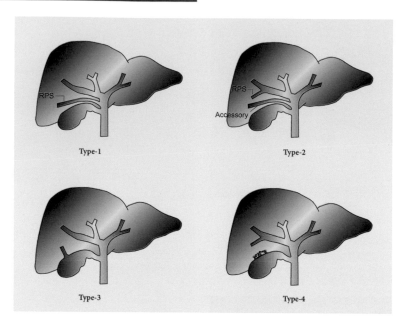

Figure 3.25 Pictorial depiction of types of subvesicle duct. *Source:* Schnelldorfer T, Sarr MG, Adams DB. *Journal of Gastrointestinal Surgery* 2012; 16:656–662.

Subvesicle duct, located in close proximity to the GB bed, is present in 34.5% of cases.[1] A more recent review, however, reported an incidence of 3%–10%.[2] The mean diameter of the duct is usually less than 2 mm. Four types of ducts have been identified (Figures 3.25–3.27).

Type 1: A segmental or sectoral duct: Right posterior segmental (RPS) duct that runs close to gallbladder bed to join the main duct.

Type 2: An accessary duct: Arising from the right anterior or posterior segmental duct, and drains into the main duct.

Type 3: Cholecystohepatic duct: The duct drains into the gallbladder.

Type 4: A series of minute ducts that end blindly in the connective tissue of the gallbladder bed.

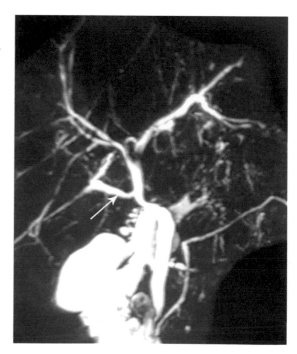

Figure 3.26 MRCP showing right posterior sectoral duct (arrow) joining common hepatic duct below the hilar confluence close to the cystic duct insertion.

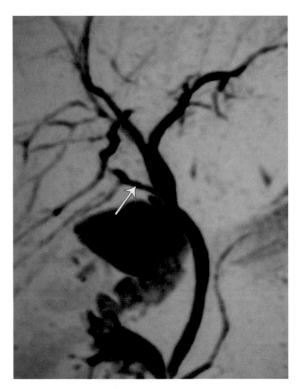

Figure 3.27 MRCP showing right posterior sectoral duct (arrow) joining common hepatic duct below the hilar confluence close to the cystic duct insertion.

CYSTIC ARTERY

The cystic artery arises from the right hepatic artery and crosses the hepatocystic (HC) triangle to supply the gallbladder in approximately 80% of cases. In the remaining, it can arise from any named branch of the celiac trunk i.e. common hepatic artery, left or middle hepatic artery, gastroduodenal artery or directly from the main trunk itself (Fig 3.28). Its course in the HC triangle varies depending on its origin. In nearly 20%, the cystic artery remains outside the HC triangle. At the gallbladder neck it divides into superficial and deep branches. The superficial branch runs on the anterior surface of the gallbladder. The deep branch runs in the gallbladder bed. Multiple cystic arteries, ranging from two to four, have been reported in 9% with each originating from different vessels. Alternatively, an early division into superficial and deep branches and also branches to infundibulum and cystic duct can give an impression of multiple cystic arteries (Figs 3.29–3.36). The cystic artery is usually short (<1 cm) and may comprise of several minor branches when it arises from an aberrant or tortuous right hepatic artery coursing close to the gallbladder surface. The cystic artery may be absent in 0.3%. The position of the cystic artery in relation to CBD is shown in Table 3.2 and the anomalies of RHA in Figures 3.37 and 3.38.

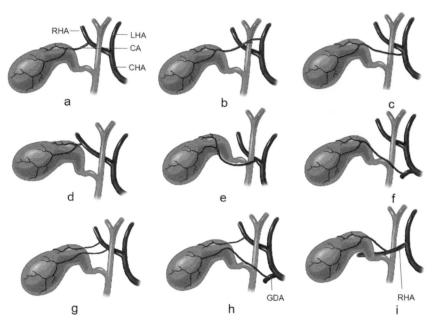

Figure 3.28 Commonly encountered origin and position of cystic artery. **(a)** Normal disposition of CA from RHA, **(b)** CA from LHA and anterior to CHD, **(c)** CA from CHA anterior to CBD, **(d)** RHA hump with short CA, **(e)** CA from RHA and anterior to CBD, **(f)** CA arising from GDA, **(g)** Double CA from RHA, **(h)** Double CA from RHA and GDA, **(i)** Aberrant RHA. *Source:* Adapted from: Andall RG, Matusz P, du Plessis M et al. *Surgical Radiological Anatomy* 2016; 38: 529–39.

Table 3.2 Position of cystic artery

Position of the cystic artery with respect to cystic duct (CD), common bile duct (CBD) and common hepatic duct (CHD)			
Position	CD (%)	CBD (%)	CHD (%)
Anterior	33.8	5.4	17.9
Posterior	12.8	3.9	10.3
Inferior	4.9	2.9	10.3
Superior	15.2	-	28.6
To the left	2.9	-	4.5
To the right	1.7	-	29.7

Source: Andall RG, Matusz P, du Plessis M et al. *Surgical Radiological Anatomy* 2016; 38: 529–39.

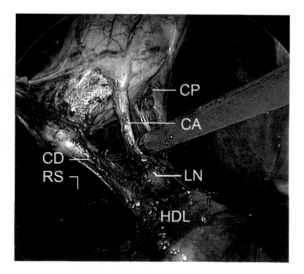

Figure 3.29 Single cystic artery in the hepatocystic triangle after dissection. This is the most common type of anatomy.

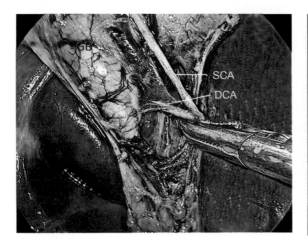

Figure 3.30 Cystic artery having clearly identified superficial and deep branches. The superficial branch supplies the gallbladder neck region and the deep branch run towards the body.

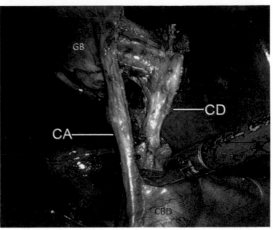

Figure 3.32 Low cystic artery: Cystic artery is lying postero-inferior to the cystic duct. This anatomical relationship is seen when the cystic artery origi-nates from the gastroduodenal artery.

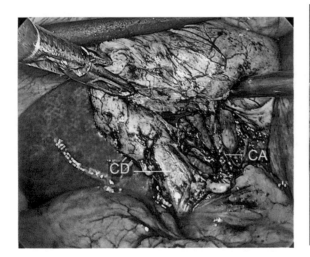

Figure 3.31 Cystic artery dividing into superficial and deep branches early in its course in the hepatocystic triangle. Note the wide cystic duct.

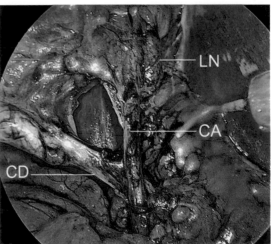

Figure 3.33 Cystic artery arising inferior to the cystic duct and passing anteriorly to enter the hepatocystic triangle.

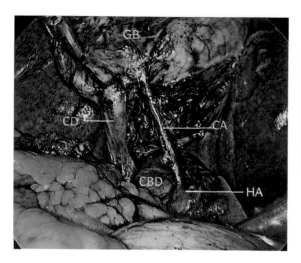

Figure 3.34 The cystic artery is crossing the common bile duct to enter the hepatocystic triangle. The origin of the cystic artery is medial to CBD from the hepatic artery.

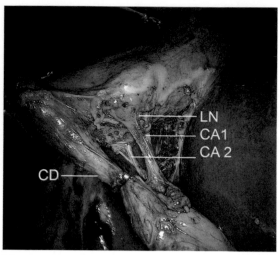

(a)

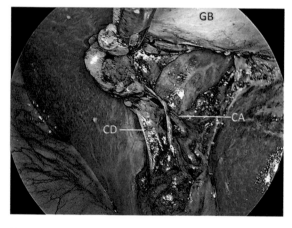

Figure 3.35 A short cystic artery along with multiple twigs supplying the cystic duct and gallbladder.

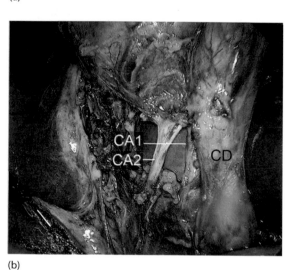

(b)

Figure 3.36 Double cystic artery. **(a)** Anterior view – Two cystic arteries in the hepatocystic triangle. **(b)** Posterior view – Note the arteries arising in two different planes indicating their different sources of origin. Cystic duct is dilated.

RIGHT HEPATIC ARTERY

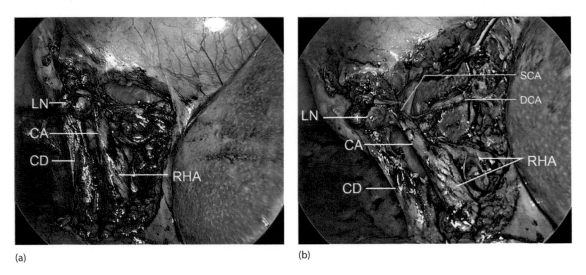

(a)   (b)

Figure 3.37 Right hepatic artery hump. **(a)** An artery running alongside the cystic duct is seen on initial dissection of the hepatocystic triangle. **(b)** On further dissection, it is identified as the right hepatic artery coursing close to gallbladder (caterpillar hump). A short cystic artery is seen arising from it and subsequently bifurcating into superficial and deep branches.

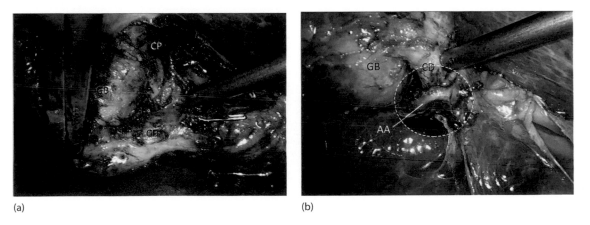

(a)   (b)

Figure 3.38 Aberrant right hepatic artery. **(a)** No proper cystic artery is found during dissection of gallbladder infundibulum and distal body. **(b)** An aberrant vessel, possibly right hepatic or a segmental artery, is seen crossing the cystic duct and inserting into the gallbladder bed.

HEPATOCYSTIC TRIANGLE AND 'CRITICAL VIEW OF SAFETY'

Calot's triangle is traditionally considered important for cholecystectomy. It is bound by the common hepatic duct, cystic artery and cystic duct (Fig 3.39). The hepatocystic triangle, which is more relevant to safe cholecystectomy, is bound by the common hepatic duct, gallbladder and liver surface in the GB bed. Configuration of this triangle changes with dissection (Fig 3.40). Meticulous dissection of this triangle is the *most important* step in cholecystectomy and the key to achieving the 'Critical View of Safety' (CVS). The three components that define CVS are:

i. Hepatocystic triangle cleared of all fibro-fatty tissue
ii. Dissected gallbladder to expose the lower one-third of the cystic plate and

iii. Demonstration of *two and only two* structures i.e. cystic duct and artery entering the gallbladder. (Figs 3.41 and 3.42)

Clearance of the hepatocystic triangle and the exposure of the cystic plate essentially serves to reveal any aberrant bilio-vascular anatomy which, if undetected, may jeopardise the safety of cholecystectomy.

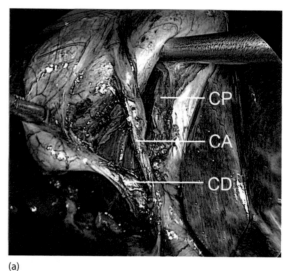

(a)

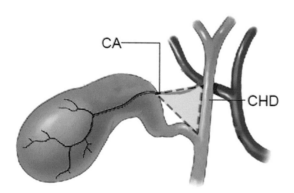

Figure 3.39 Calot's triangle.

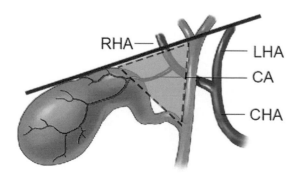

Figure 3.40 Hepatocystic triangle.

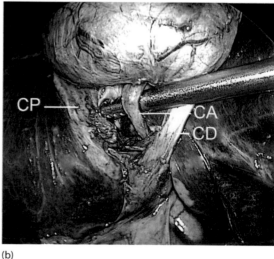

(b)

Figure 3.41 CVS **(a)** Anterior view, **(b)** Posterior view. Single cystic artery and cystic duct displayed after clearing the hepatocystic triangle. The distal body of the gallbladder has been dissected off the cystic plate.

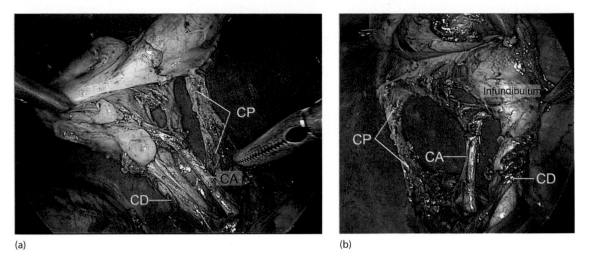

(a) (b)

Figure 3.42 CVS: **(a)**. anterior view, **(b)**. posterior view. Note cystic artery dividing into superficial and deep branches near the infundibulum.

NOTES

1 Vakili K, Pomfret EA. Biliary Anatomy and Embryology. *Surgical Clinics of North America.* 2008; 88: 1159–1174.
2 Schnelldorfer T, Sarr MG, Adams DB. *Journal of Gastrointestinal Surgery* 2012; 16:656–662.

4

Steps of Laparoscopic Cholecystectomy and the 'Critical View of Safety'

The basic principles and the steps of surgery are primarily aimed at the safe removal of the gallbladder, with no complications and without injury to the bile duct. Demonstrating the 'Critical View of Safety' (CVS) is undeniably the most reproducible method to prevent bilio-vascular injury following laparoscopic cholecystectomy.

Overview

- Equipment checks
- Pneumoperitoneum and port placement
- Proper retraction of the gallbladder
- Identification of operative landmarks and dissection planes
- Achieving CVS
- Alternative techniques when CVS cannot be achieved
- Ligation/clipping and division of the cystic artery and duct
- Other safety measures
- Dissection of the gallbladder and extraction
- Removal of ports and fascial closure

Equipment:

- High-definition camera with a 30° telescope is preferred, as this provides a clear view of the hepatocystic triangle for safe dissection during cholecystectomy.

- Diathermy
  - Co-axially shielded instruments
  - Use blend current
  - Low diathermy setting <30 W
  - Use bipolar cautery during dissection
- An ultrasonic coagulator (Harmonic scalpel) can prove useful in specific situations.

Pneumoperitoneum and port placement (Fig 4.1):

- Open pneumoperitoneum through the umbilical (camera) port is preferred.
- Lateral traction port (3 mm or 5 mm) is placed in the anterior axillary line.
- Working ports - epigastric port (5 mm) and mid-axillary line port (3 mm or 5 mm), are positioned to ensure triangulation and 90-degree access to the hepatocystic triangle. A 10 mm epigastric port instead of 5 mm, may be placed for using conventional clip applicator.

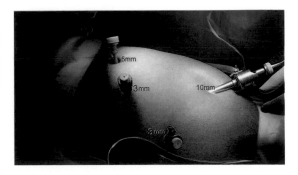

Figure 4.1 Port placement for laparoscopic cholecystectomy.

DOI: 10.1201/9781003174547-4

Proper retraction of the gallbladder:

- Retraction of the fundus and Hartman's pouch is important to lay open the hepatocystic triangle. The fundus of the gallbladder should be retracted cranially towards the right shoulder (10 o'clock position) as opposed to the 12 or 1 o'clock position (Fig 4.2). It is critical that this direction of retraction is checked frequently during surgery since it often tends to move more medially (12 o'clock).
- The Hartman's pouch (infundibulum) is retracted infero-laterally so as to open up the hepatocystic triangle and also to place the cystic duct out of alignment with the common bile duct. This prevents the misidentification of the common bile duct as the cystic duct.
- Pericholecystic adhesions are brought down and operative landmarks are displayed. During adhesiolysis, care must be taken to prevent injury to any adherent hollow viscera like duodenum and colon.

Identification of operative landmarks and dissection planes (*refer to Chapter 3 for details*):

- Rouviere's sulcus is an important landmark. The plane of dissection should remain above the R4U line.
- The plane of falciform ligament marks the medial most margin of the bilio-vascular structures in the hepatoduodenal ligament. Hence, dissection must remain lateral to it.
- Cystic lymph node marks the location of the cystic artery.
- Supero-lateral quadrant (shaded in Figure 4.3) of the intersection of cystic lymph node line & R4U line is considered the safe zone for dissection.
- After retraction of the gallbladder as mentioned above, a visual impression is made about structures in the hepatoduodenal ligament, i.e., common bile duct and cystic duct and artery.
- Incise the posterior peritoneum to release the gallbladder, which opens up the hepatocystic triangle anteriorly for dissection and the identification of critical structures (Fig 4.4).

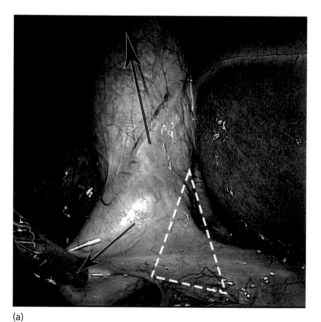

(a)

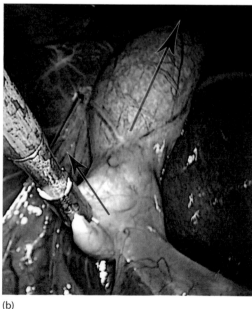

(b)

Figure 4.2 **(a)** Correct retraction of the gallbladder to expose hepatocystic triangle, **(b)** Incorrect retraction of gallbladder.

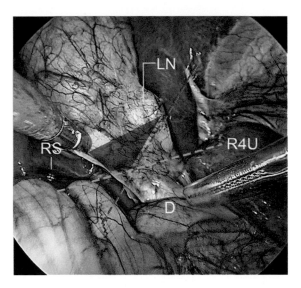

Figure 4.3 Anatomical landmarks and planes for safe dissection. Supero-lateral quadrant (shaded area) is considered the 'safe zone'.

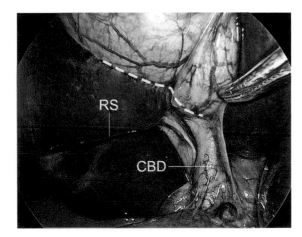

Figure 4.4 Incision on posterior peritoneum (dotted line) to start dissection.

Achieving CVS:

- The hepatocystic triangle is cleared of all fibro-fatty tissue.
- Distal third of the gallbladder is dissected off the cystic plate; so that any aberrant duct or artery in relation to gallbladder is identified and protected.

- Two structures, i.e., the cystic duct and the cystic artery, are clearly displayed joining the gallbladder.
- After achieving CVS, an intraoperative 'time-out' and documenting 'doublet-view' (photographing anterior and posterior view of CVS) should be done (Fig 4.5).
- Cystic artery may need to be clipped and divided early in some situations to facilitate the clearing of the hepatocystic triangle. In that case the artery should be divided lateral to the cystic lymph node close to the gallbladder wall. Division of the cystic duct, however, must always be done after the proper delineation of CVS.

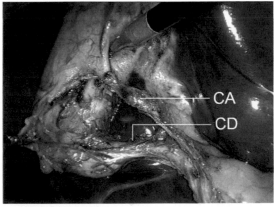

(a)

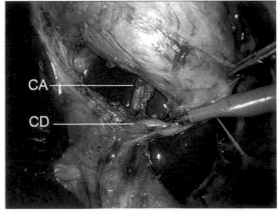

(b)

Figure 4.5 'Critical View of Safety': **(a)** anterior view, **(b)** posterior view.

Alternative techniques when CVS cannot be achieved:

In a subset of patients, it may not be possible to achieve CVS due to acute inflammation, chronic fibrosis or unclear anatomy. The following alternative strategies should be considered in these situations.

- Cholecystectomy by antegrade (fundus-first) technique
- Subtotal cholecystectomy
- Cholecystostomy
- Conversion to open cholecystectomy.

Refer to specific chapters for detailed management of cystic duct, cystic artery, gallbladder bed and alternative techniques.

Other safety measures:

- Avoid excessive lateral and cranial traction on gallbladder fundus. The liver at falciform attachment may tear and bleed (Fig 4.6).
- DO NOT use excessive cautery during dissection of the hepatocystic triangle.
- In case of any unexpected bleeding, give pressure; identify the bleeding source and control. Do not apply clips blindly or do mass cauterization of the tissues.
- Any bile staining in the operative field requires careful inspection, identification of the source and appropriate action

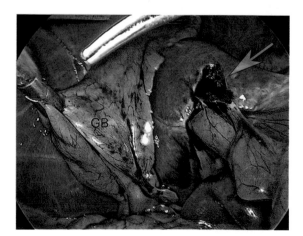

Figure 4.6 Tear at the base of falciform ligament (arrow) resulting from excessive cranial traction on fundus.

Dissection of the gallbladder and extraction:

- Gallbladder is dissected from the liver bed, (Fig 4.7a) preserving the cystic plate
- Hemostasis is secured in the gallbladder bed
- Any spilled stones are retrieved and collected in a bag
- Gallbladder is parked in the retrieval bag (Fig 4.7b) and extracted through the umbilical port. This prevents spillage of stones and contamination of the extraction port with infected bile and spilled stones.

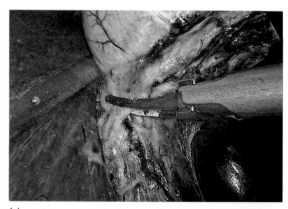

(a)

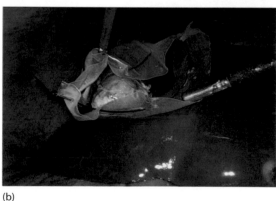

(b)

Figure 4.7 **(a)** Gallbladder dissection from liver bed. **(b)** Retrieval bag (endobag) containing gall bladder after its removal.

Removal of Ports:

- Final inspection of the operative site is done
- All ports are removed under vision
- Umbilical port fascial closure is done under vision

STEPS OF SAFE CHOLECYSTECTOMY

The following illustrative cases present the steps of surgery to achieve complete CVS in presence of normal and variant anatomy.

CVS in Presence of Normal Anatomy (1): Video v1

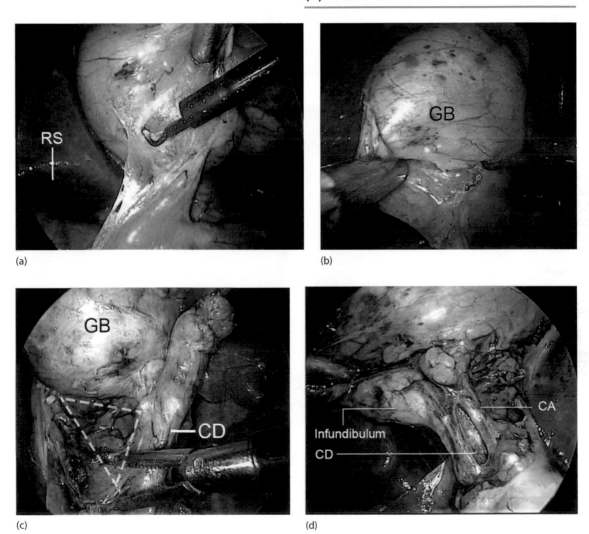

(a) (b)

(c) (d)

Figure 4.8 **(a)** The Hartman's pouch is retracted towards the left to expose Rouviere's sulcus. The posterior peritoneum is incised with an L hook close to the gallbladder wall. **(b)** The anterior peritoneum is incised, which is extended up along the anterior wall of the gallbladder. This is the preliminary step to expose and dissect the hepatocystic triangle. **(c)** Posterior dissection – Fibro-fatty tissue in the hepatocystic triangle (dotted triangle) is cleared. **(d)** Anterior dissection exposing the cystic duct and artery.

(Continued)

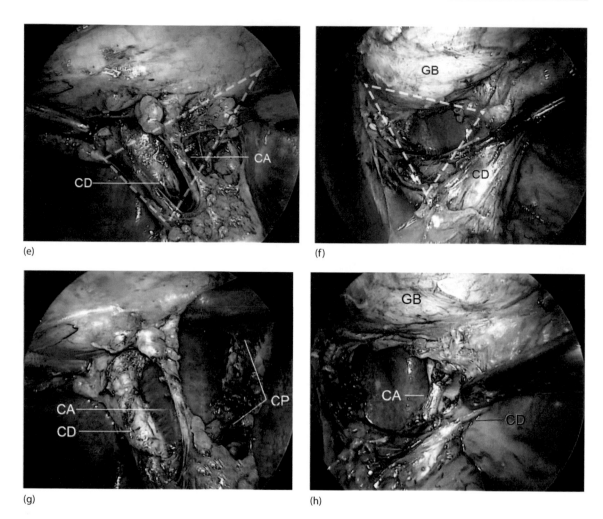

(e)

(f)

(g)

(h)

Figure 4.8 (Continued) **(e)** As dissection progresses in the hepatocystic triangle (dotted triangle), the cystic duct and artery come into view. **(f)** Posterior view – the window created after the clearance of fibro-fatty tissue. The dissection is carried up further (dotted triangle) to mobilise the body of the gallbladder off the cystic plate. The hepatocystic triangle is completely cleared and the body of the gallbladder is dissected off the cystic plate, thus establishing CVS. **(g)** Anterior view. **(h)** Posterior view.

CVS in Presence of Normal Anatomy (2)

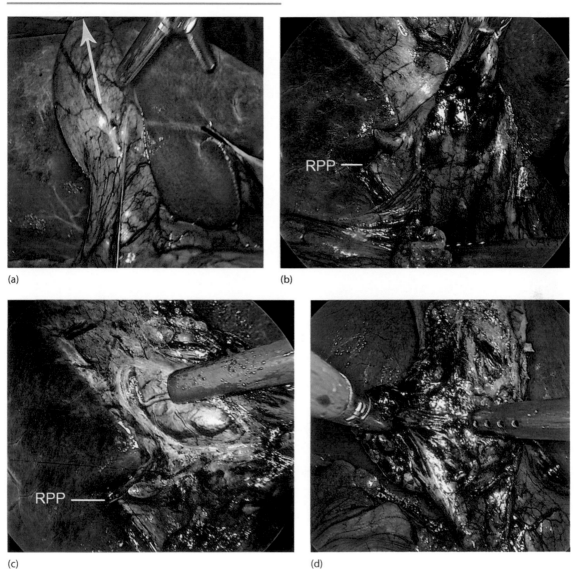

(a)

(b)

(c)

(d)

Figure 4.9 **(a)** Gallbladder is retracted (in the direction of arrow) for inspection. **(b)** Posterior surface is exposed by retracting Hartman's pouch towards the left. Rouviere's sulcus is absent. However, a notch indicating right portal pedicle corresponds to the plane of RS. **(c)** Posterior peritoneum is incised and incision extended upwards. **(d)** Anteriorly, peritoneum over the hepatocystic triangle is incised.

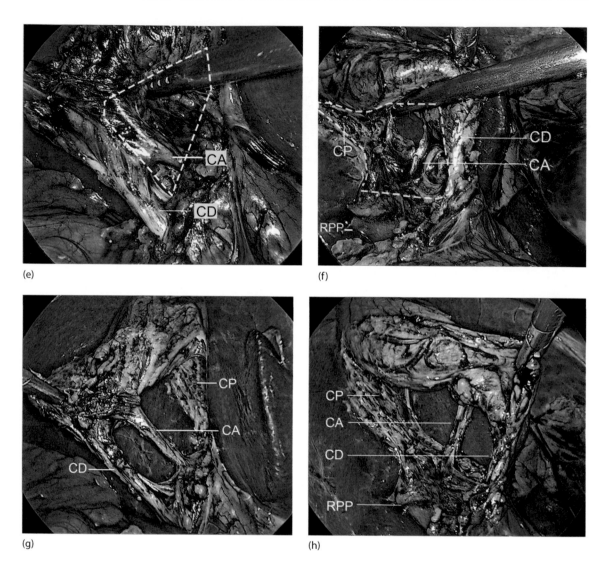

(e) (f)

(g) (h)

Figure 4.9 (Continued) **(e)** On further dissection, the cystic duct and artery are identified. The dotted area marks the hepatocystic triangle that is to be dissected to achieve CVS. **(f)** Posterior dissection in progress. Dotted lines represent the desired area of posterior dissection. In the course of dissection and clearance of fibro-fatty tissue, a window is created thus clearing the hepatocystic triangle. CVS achieved as dissection is completed. **(g)** Anterior view. **(h)** Posterior view.

CVS in Presence of Low (Anterior) Cystic Artery: Video v3

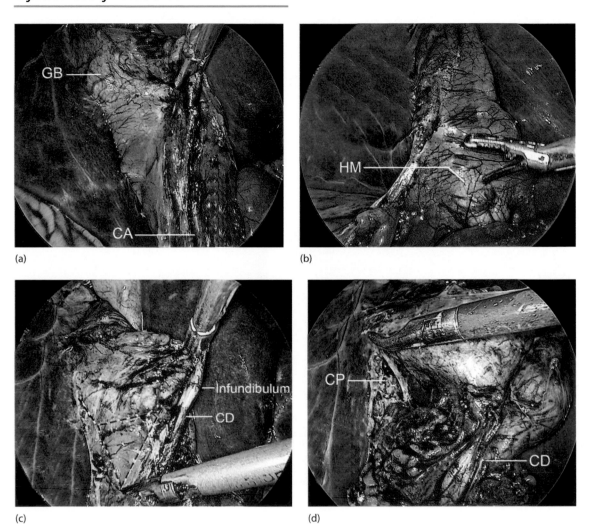

(a)

(b)

(c)

(d)

Figure 4.10 **(a).** Gallbladder and hepatoduodenal ligament are covered in a fatty layer obscuring any visible landmark. Rouviere's sulcus is absent. Note the low cystic artery visible in the fat layer. **(b)** Hartman's pouch comes into view after adhesiolysis. **(c)** Hartman's pouch is retracted towards left for posterior dissection (area marked by dotted lines). **(d)** The body of gallbladder is mobilized from the cystic plate. Note the window after dissection in the hepatocystic triangle. *(Continued)*

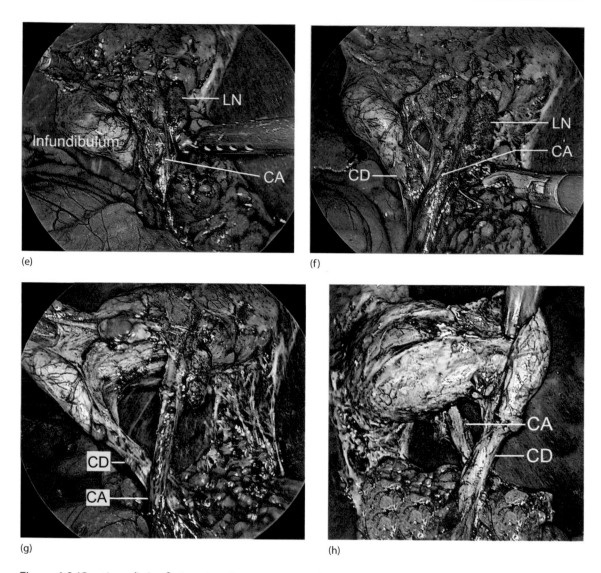

(e)

(f)

(g)

(h)

Figure 4.9 (Continued) **(e, f)** Anterior dissection. Note the cystic artery arising below the cystic duct and crossing it anteriorly. **(g)** Complete CVS – anterior view. The hepatocystic triangle is cleared of all fibro-fatty tissue. The cystic artery is crossing the cystic duct. Lymph node is adherent to artery near gallbladder surface. **(h)** CVS- posterior view.

CVS in Presence of Low (Posterior) Cystic Artery: Video v4

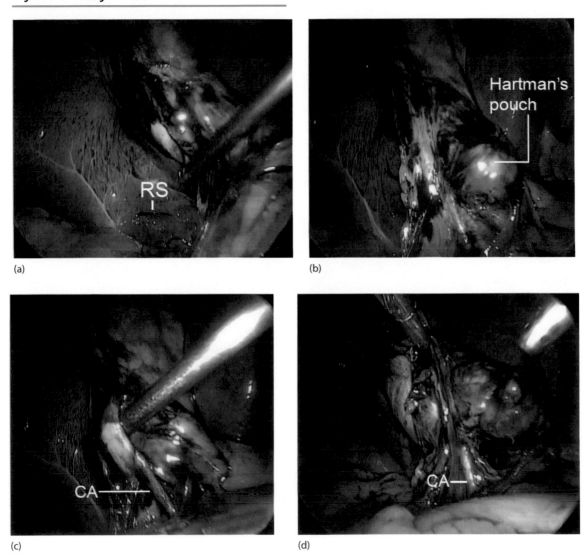

Figure 4.11 **(a)** Gallbladder is retracted towards the left for posterior dissection. **(b)** A band of fibro-fatty tissue is running from the hepatoduodenal ligament towards the posterior surface of the gallbladder. **(c)** The cystic artery appearing as a bowstring can be identified within that band of tissue. **(d)** The artery is further dissected and traced towards the posterior surface of the gallbladder. (*Continued*)

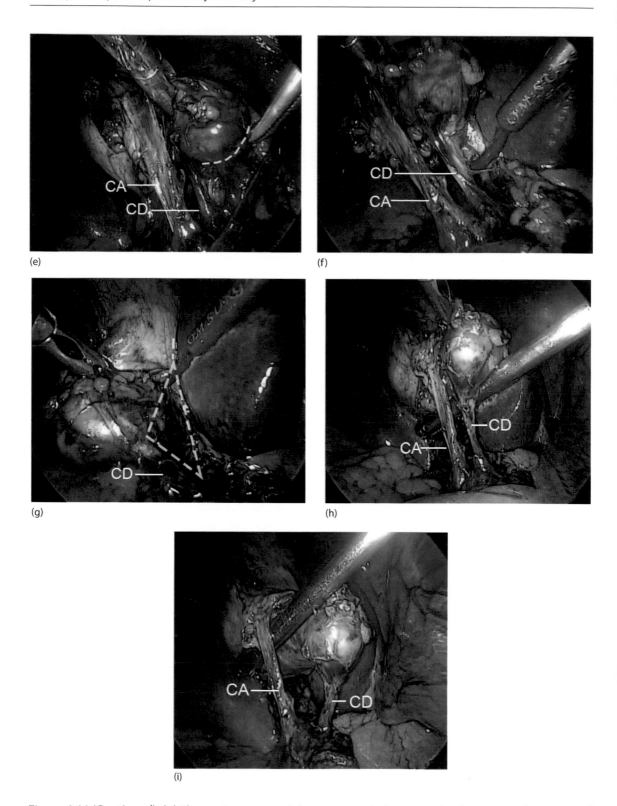

Figure 4.11 (Continued) (e) The cystic artery and duct, as seen during posterior dissection. The proposed anterior dissection is close to the Hartman's pouch (dotted line). (f) As the dissection progresses, the cystic duct and artery are better defined. (g) The dotted area marks the boundaries of the hepatocystic triangle and the extent of anterior dissection. (h) CVS – anterior view. (i) Posterior view of CVS. Note the position and course of the cystic artery.

Summary: Ten Steps of Safe Laparoscopic Cholecystectomy

1. High-definition camera, 30° telescope and a good camera operator.
2. Open pneumoperitoneum and port placement.
3. Traction of gallbladder:
   a. 10 o'clock position (towards the right shoulder).
   b. Lateral and downward traction of the Hartman's pouch.
4. Identify Rouviere's sulcus and other landmarks.
5. Open the posterior peritoneum to provide mobility to gallbladder and to open the hepatocystic triangle.
6. Define safe area of dissection and achieve the CVS.
7. Time out:
   a. Review the landmarks and anatomy.
   b. Confirm the same with the team/senior colleague.
8. Clip and divide the cystic artery and the cystic duct.
9. Dissect gallbladder from the liver bed and place in a pouch.
10. Remove ports and close fascial layer.

5

Management of the Cystic Artery and Its Variations

In nearly 80%, the cystic artery is located in the hepatocystic triangle. However, its number and course can be variable as highlighted in chapter 3. Injury to the cystic artery can result in significant bleeding, leading to conversion from laparoscopic to open cholecystectomy in about 0.1% of cases. Careful dissection, identification and division of the artery is therefore an important step in performing safe cholecystectomy.

Issues related to the cystic artery

- In approximately one-quarter of cases, the cystic artery may not be found in the hepatocystic triangle. Identification of artery in such cases requires careful dissection.
- In the case of a double cystic artery, the second artery is vulnerable to injury if not anticipated or carefully dissected.
- A tortuous or aberrant right hepatic artery is prone to be mistaken for the cystic artery with possible adverse consequences if clipped and divided inadvertently.

Operative Tips

- Knowledge of the arterial variations during cholecystectomy is important to prevent bleeding complications and to avoid injury to major vessels like the RHA.
- During the process of establishing the CVS, dissect vessels close to the gallbladder away from the hepatoduodenal ligament.
- Clip and divide vessels close to the gallbladder, even if it involves clipping multiple vessels.
- Preserve the deep branch during dissection of the gallbladder bed, as it may be a more significant segmental artery.

STANDARD MANAGEMENT

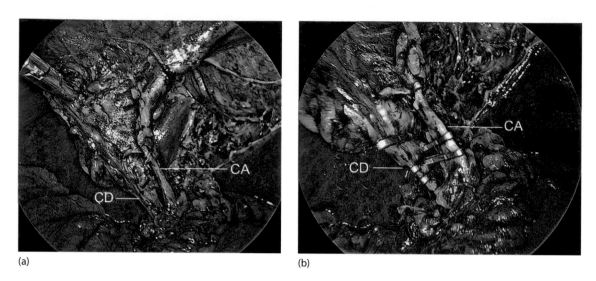

(a) (b)

Figure 5.1 **(a)** Hepatocystic triangle is dissected to isolate the cystic artery until its point of entry into the gallbladder. **(b)** Two appropriate size clips are applied proximally and one distally (towards gallbladder).

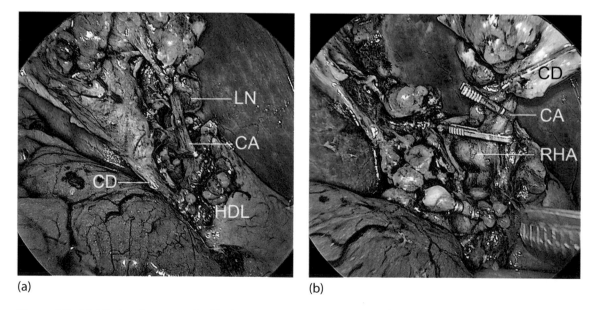

(a) (b)

Figure 5.2 **(a)** Clip has been applied below cystic artery bifurcation. **(b)** Posterior view of the artery after the division of the cystic duct. Note that the proximal clip is quite close to the right hepatic artery. This highlights the fact that the clipping of the cystic artery should be as close to the gallbladder as possible so as to avoid injury to the right hepatic artery.

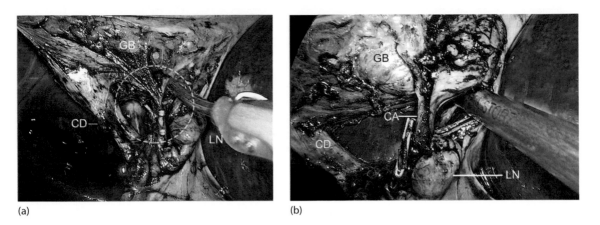

(a)   (b)

Figure 5.3 **(a, b)** Multiple minor arterial branches in the hepatocystic triangle (dotted circle) are clipped and divided before the main cystic artery is isolated.

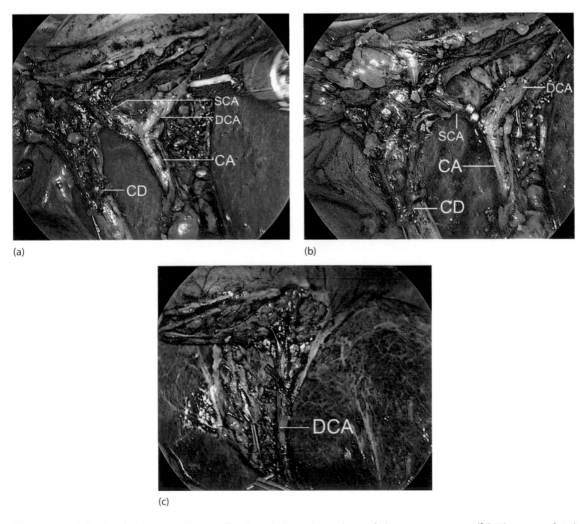

(a)   (b)

(c)

Figure 5.4 **(a)** Clearly dissected superficial and deep branches of the cystic artery. **(b)** The superficial branch (not the main cystic artery) is clipped and divided. The deep branch, because of its significant size, is traced further. **(c)** On further dissection, the deep branch is seen entering into gallbladder fundus. **(d)** It is clipped at that point and divided. (Video v5)

EARLY DIVISION OF THE CYSTIC ARTERY

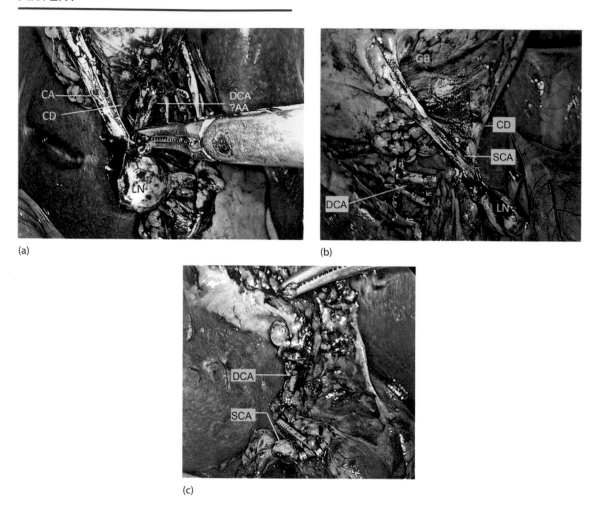

Figure 5.5 **(a, b)** Two divisions of cystic artery, superficial and deep branches, have been isolated on either side of the cystic duct. **(c)** The superficial branch is clipped and divided. The deep branch seen entering into the liver is preserved. Note the large calibre of the artery. The possibility of it being a segmental artery cannot be ruled out.

RIGHT HEPATIC ARTERY HUMP:
Video v6

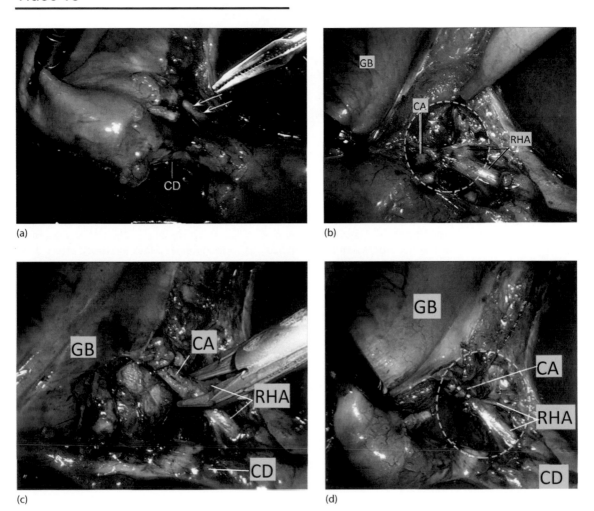

(a)

(b)

(c)

(d)

Figure 5.6 **(a)** Initial dissection of the hepatocystic triangle reveals a possible cystic artery (arrows). **(b)** On subsequent dissection, it is proved to be the right hepatic artery (caterpillar hump), giving off a small cystic artery close to the gallbladder. **(c)** The cystic artery is defined further till its entry into the gallbladder. **(d)** Two clips are applied proximally. The distal part is coagulated using bipolar cautery and divided.

(*Continued*)

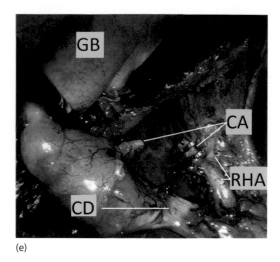

(e)

Figure 5.6 (Continued) **(e)** The divided cystic artery with RHA is clearly identified. *The above case highlights the need to dissect the hepatocystic triangle meticulously, define and isolate the cystic artery close to the gallbladder before clipping and division.*

6

Management of the Cystic Duct

An important component of laparoscopic cholecystectomy constitutes the proper identification, isolation, ligation/clipping and division of the cystic duct. Mismanagement of the cystic duct can result in a host of complications, ranging from bile leak to common bile duct injury and eventually formation of stricture. Length, calibre and contents of the cystic duct and its course each require individual attention and appropriate management.

STANDARD MANAGEMENT OF THE CYSTIC DUCT

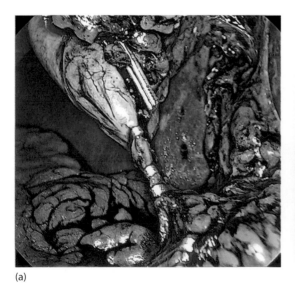

(a)

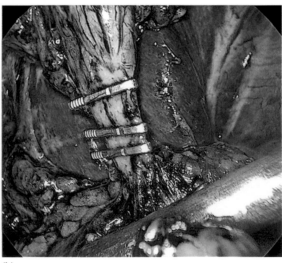

(b)

Figure 6.1 Standard management of the cystic duct: **(a)** Anterior view. **(b)** Posterior view. Two clips of appropriate size are placed distally and one clip proximally (towards the gallbladder). Ideally, the clips should completely cover the duct and project beyond. The duct is divided after making sure to leave a rim of tissue beyond the distal clip. This would provide adequate stability to the clips against accidental slippage.

DOI: 10.1201/9781003174547-6

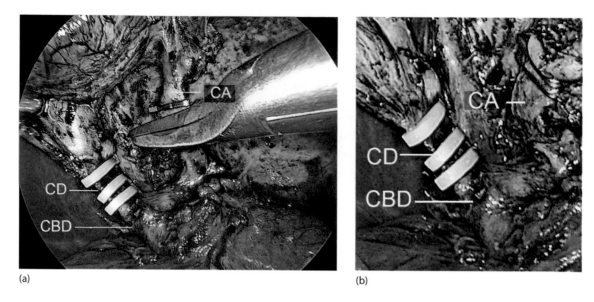

(a)

(b)

Figure 6.2 Angulated common bile duct: Anterior view. **(a, b)** Common duct appearing angulated due to excessive traction on the gallbladder and cystic duct. Hem-o-lok clips have, however, been safely placed away from the angulation. These nonabsorbable polymer locking clips are considered more secure than the metal clips. *It is always a good and safe practice to release traction on the gallbladder and cystic duct while applying the distal-most clip and ensuring that there is no encroachment on the lumen of the CBD.*

WIDE CYSTIC DUCT

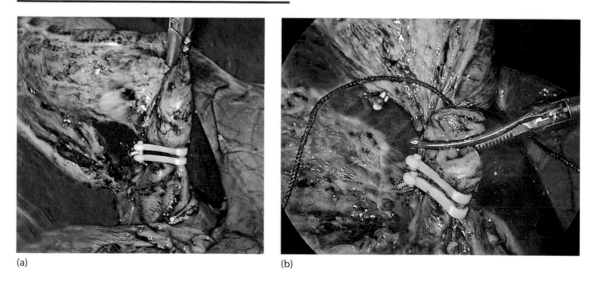

(a)

(b)

Figure 6.3 **(a)** Any possible stone in the dilated cystic duct must be milked back into the gallbladder. **(b)** After placing the clips (Hem-o-lok preferably), a ligature can be applied to occlude the proximal end before the cystic duct is divided.

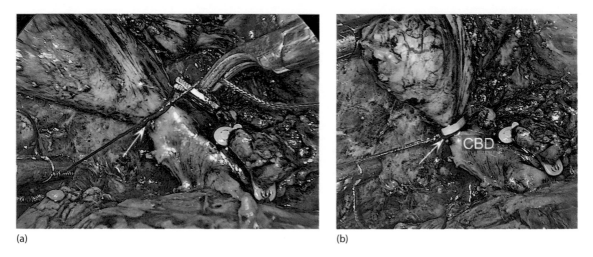

(a)

(b)

Figure 6.4 **(a)** Dilated and effaced cystic duct that is difficult to secure even with a large clip. The infundibulum is encircled and ligated with a 2–0 Vicryl suture (arrow). **(b)** The ligature constricts the infundibulum allowing the placement of a Hem-o-lok (arrow) clip that is *hitherto* not possible. Doubly secured by the ligature and the clip, the infundibulum is divided, leaving behind an adequate cuff.

ABSENT OR UNIDENTIFIABLE CYSTIC DUCT

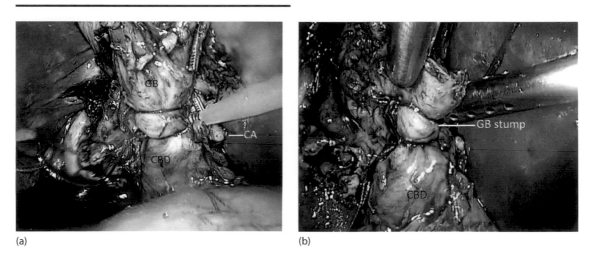

(a)

(b)

Figure 6.5 Sessile gallbladder: Inflammatory obliteration of the cystic duct has resulted in the appearance of a sessile gallbladder. The cystic duct can be appreciated as a groove at the gallbladder and the common bile duct junction. **(a)** The gallbladder is mobilized circumferentially by fundus-first technique. At a safe distance from the common bile duct, the infundibulum is doubly ligated with Vicryl suture. **(b)** The gallbladder is excised leaving behind at least half cm long cuff.

CYSTIC DUCT INJURY

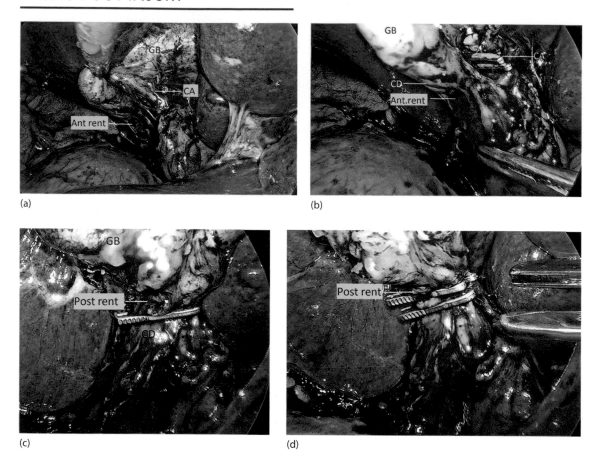

(a)

(b)

(c)

(d)

Figure 6.6 Rent in the cystic duct: **(a)** During the dissection of the cystic duct an accidental rent is detected on the anterior as well as the posterior aspect of the cystic duct. The anterior rent is a longitudinal tear with mucosal breach at the apex. **(b)** Free flow of golden yellow bile indicates its proximity to common bile duct. **(c, d)** Two large-sized clips are satisfactorily positioned beyond the rent without compromising the common bile duct lumen.

CYSTIC DUCT STONE/S

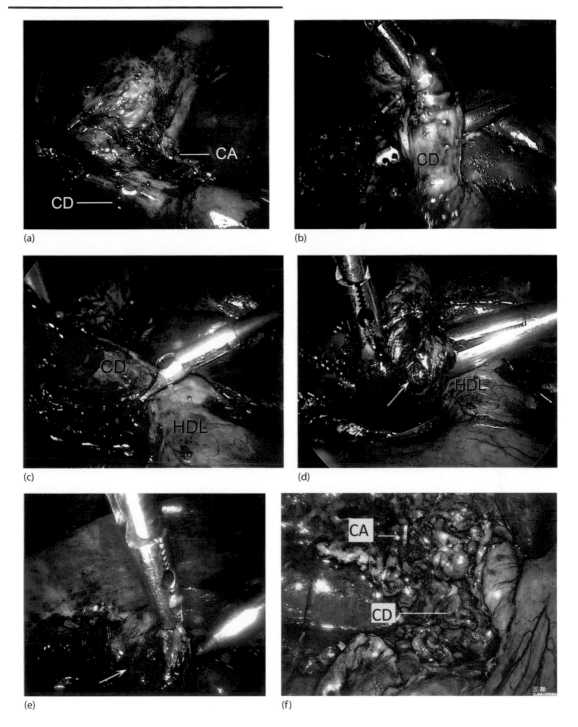

Figure 6.7 (a) The cystic duct is dilated due to the presence of multiple stones. **(a)** Dissected and mobilized cystic duct. **(c)** The cystic duct is milked to displace stones into the gallbladder. **(d)** The duct is partially incised to extract the stones (arrow). **(e)** The cystic duct is divided and irrigated with normal saline and its lumen (arrow) inspected for any leftover stone or debris. **(f)** The stump is doubly secured with endoloop and the cholecystectomy is completed.

7

Management of the Gallbladder Bed

The removal of the gallbladder from its bed is the last major step in cholecystectomy. The gallbladder bed comprises of a fibrous layer, the 'cystic plate', that overlies the liver parenchyma. The space between the gallbladder and the cystic plate is traversed by fibro-areolar tissue, blood vessels and lymphatics. In the absence of any major inflammation, this layer is well preserved and can be easily dissected without blood loss (Fig 7.1). Chronic inflammation renders it fibrotic, resulting in firm adhesions between the gallbladder and the cystic plate. Dissection under such circumstances can result in either the perforation of the gallbladder, leading to bile and stone spillage, or a breach of the cystic plate with the risk of serious bleeding and/or bile leak (Table 7.1).

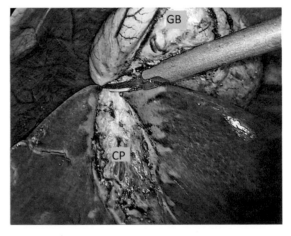

Figure 7.1 During removal of the gallbladder, the dissection plane remains superficial to the cystic plate. The intervening fibro-areolar tissue is divided using L hook or spatula or ultrasonic coagulator. The gallbladder can be removed with no or minimal blood loss if the plane of dissection is not violated.

Table 7.1 Structures at risk during dissection of the gallbladder bed

Superficial to cystic plate
Deep branch of the cystic artery
Aberrant right hepatic or segmental artery
Cholecystohepatic duct
Deep to the cystic plate
Hepatic vein tributaries
Subvesicle duct

DOI: 10.1201/9781003174547-7

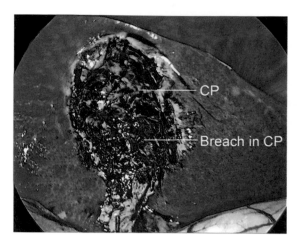

Figure 7.2 Gallbladder bed showing cystic plate as white fibrous sheet that has been breached at places due to inflammatory adhesions. Bleeding from the denuded area requires cauterization.

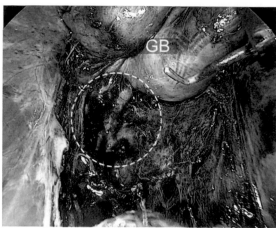

Figure 7.4 Dilated veins in the gallbladder bed (dotted circle) that has the potential for serious bleeding if injured.

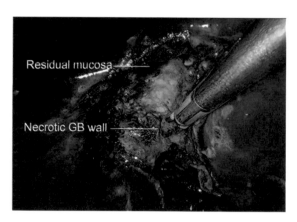

Figure 7.3 Gallbladder bed in acute gangrenous cholecystitis. The posterior wall of the gallbladder is necrotic and adherent to the bed. Gallbladder is removed, leaving behind the adherent wall. The mucosa is ablated by cauterization.

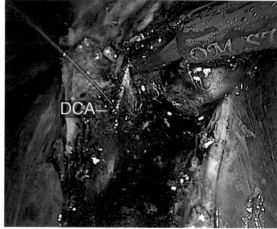

Figure 7.5 Bleeding from a deep branch of the cystic artery during dissection of the gallbladder.

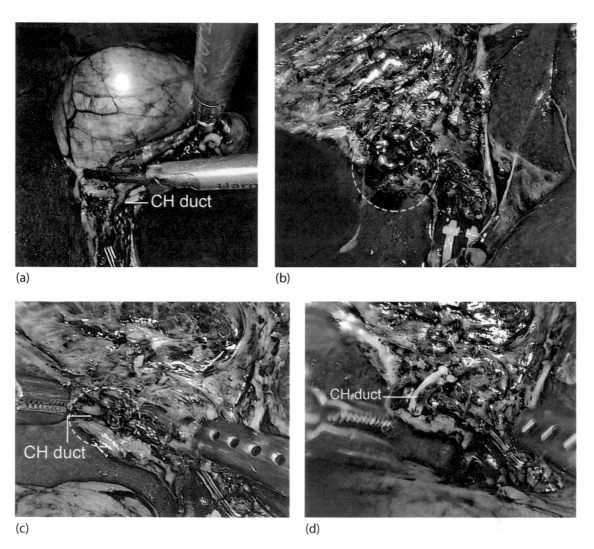

Figure 7.6 Video v8. Bile leak from gallbladder bed. **(a)** Inadvertent division of the cholecystohepatic duct during dissection of the gallbladder (retrospective identification). **(b)** Leaking duct (dotted circle) in the gallbladder bed. **(c)** The leaking duct is identified by cleaning the area with repeated suction and irrigation. **(d)** The duct is occluded with a Hem-o-lok clip.

8

Alternative Techniques in Difficult Situations

Acute, chronic or recurrent inflammation of the gallbladder, the presence of stone in the bile duct, Mirizzi's syndrome or portal hypertension can all alter the local anatomy, making the demonstration of 'Critical View of Safety' (CVS) either difficult or impossible. The following techniques can be adopted in such situations. The suitability and application of the specific technique depends on surgeon's experience and the underlying findings and pathology in the individual case.

FUNDUS-FIRST CHOLECYSTECTOMY: Video v9

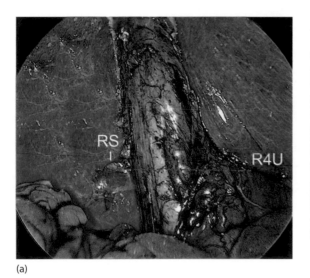

(a)

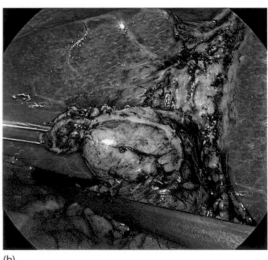

(b)

Figure 8.1 **(a)** A contracted gallbladder 'seemingly' extending down to the duodenum. Such an appearance is deceptive and calls for extreme caution and restraint. R4U line should be considered the plane to start dissection and the segment below that should be treated as the common bile duct, unless proved otherwise. The fundus-first approach is adopted when the initial trial dissection fails to delineate the hepatocystic triangle. **(b)** The fundus of the gallbladder is mobilized carefully, maintaining the dissection within the cystic plate. *(Continued)*

DOI: 10.1201/9781003174547-8

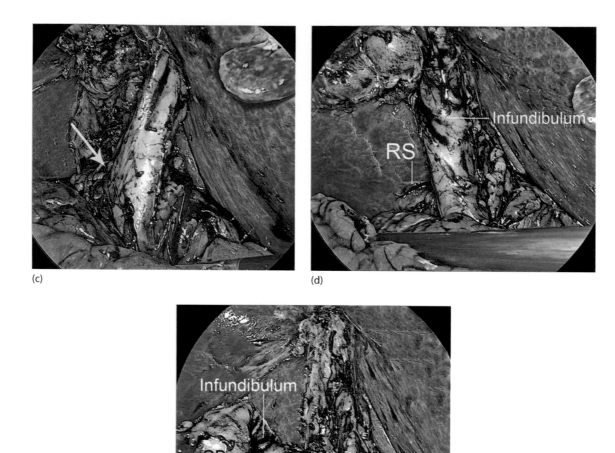

(c)

(d)

(e)

Figure 8.1 (Continued) **(c)** The gallbladder is mobilized down till hilum. Funnelling of the dissected gallbladder (arrow) indicates its junction with the common bile duct. **(d)** Alternatively, Rouviere's sulcus should serve as limit of dissection during the fundus-first approach. **(e)** Anterior view after fundal traction is released. The junction between the common duct (dotted line) and the infundibulum can be identified clearly.   (*Continued*)

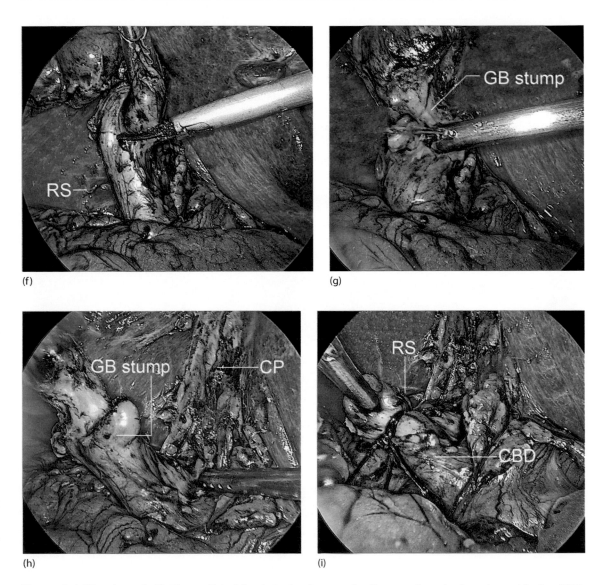

Figure 8.1 (Continued) **(f)** The gallbladder is incised at a safe distance from its junction with the CBD. **(g)** The distal remnant is irrigated with normal saline to flush out any stone or sludge. **(h)** Gallbladder is transected. **(i)** The stump was doubly ligated using endoloop. A subhepatic drain is placed.

SUBTOTAL CHOLECYSTECTOMY

Subtotal cholecystectomy is indicated for stone/s impacted in Hartman's pouch, grossly contracted gallbladder or Mirizzi's syndrome and also in situations where the hepatocystic triangle is either completely obliterated or hazardous to dissect. As a safety measure, the posterior wall of the gallbladder and/or a cuff adjacent to the bile duct is retained.

The gallbladder remnant is either suture-approximated (reconstituting type) or the cystic duct opening is closed from inside (fenestrating type).[1] The adoption of this technique in these difficult situations helps to prevent bile duct injury. Retained stone and postoperative bile leak are the two most common complications associated with subtotal cholecystectomy, with an incidence of 3.1% and 18%, respectively.[2]

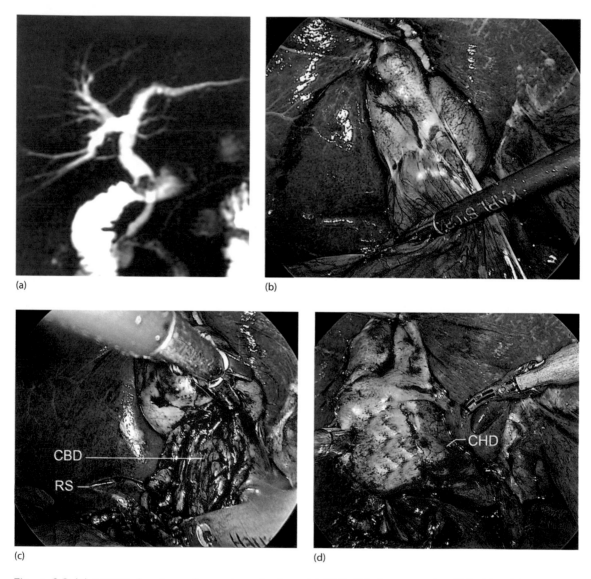

(a)   (b)   (c)   (d)

Figure 8.2 **(a)** MRCP showing a large stone in the mid-CBD. **(b)** Contracted gallbladder. **(c)** Posterior view: CBD adherent to gallbladder. (d) Anterior view: Obliterated hepatocystic triangle due to chronic inflammation.

(*Continued*)

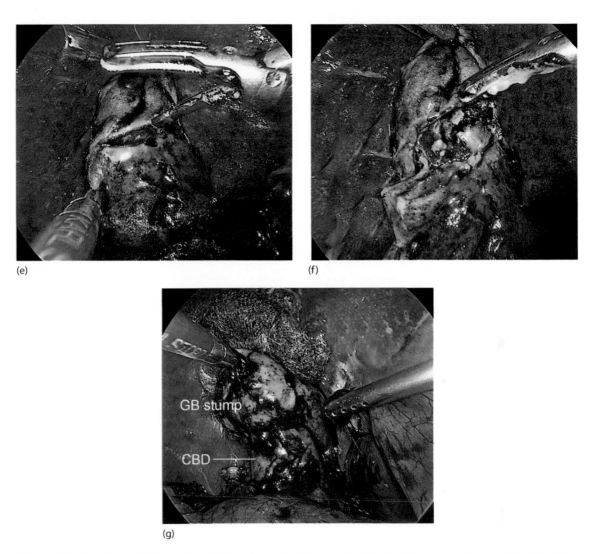

(e)

(f)

(g)

Figure 8.2 (Continued) **(e)** In view of the above findings, a decision is taken to perform subtotal chole-cystectomy. The gallbladder is incised at a safe distance from the hilum. **(f)** Stones are evacuated. **(g)** The gallbladder is bisected and the distal stump is flushed with saline to clear any stone or sludge.

(Continued)

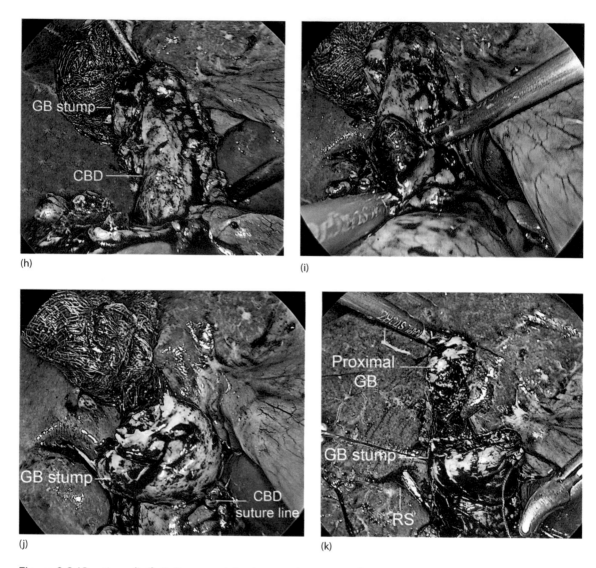

(h)

(i)

(j)

(k)

Figure 8.2 (Continued) (h,i) Common bile duct exploration and stone extraction is performed by makng an anterior choledochotomy. (j) Choledochotomy incision is closed after placing a transpapillary internal stent. (k). The gallbladder stump is closed with interrupted 2–0 Vicryl suture. The proximal stump is dissected from the gallbladder bed.

(Continued)

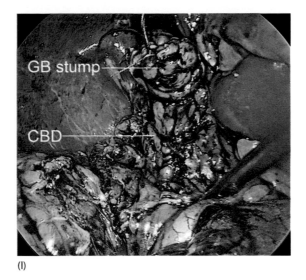

(I)

Figure 8.2 (Continued) **(I)** The gallbladder stump and the common bile duct after suture closure of both.

Fundus-first and/or sub-total cholecystectomy is a safe option in cases of obliterated anatomy, especially in the hepatocystic triangle. The most important consideration in this technique is the level of division of the gallbladder. This can be ascertained by using Rouviere's sulcus as the landmark and/or by frequent inspection of both the anterior and posterior views during dissection. In difficult situations, the GB can be divided in the middle, contents of the stump are evacuated and cleared, the lumen is inspected and further excision (revision) of the GB cuff is carried out. The key is to ensure that there are no residual stones and the GB stump is small, but adequate enough for a safe closure. Large GB stump predisposes to recurrent stone formation and symptoms. The cystic artery should be controlled at the divided margin by cautery or suture ligation. Proximal ligation of the artery may jeopardize the viability of the GB stump. A subhepatic drain must be placed in all cases undergoing subtotal cholecystectomy.

NOTES

1 Strasberg SM, Pucci MJ, Brunt LM, Deziel DJ. Subtotal Cholecystectomy – "Fenestrating" vs "Reconstituting" Subtypes and the Prevention of Bile Duct Injury: Definition of the Optimal Procedure in Difficult Operative Conditions. *Journal of American College of Surgeons.* 2016; 222: 89-96.
2 Elshaer M, Gravante G, Thomas K et al. Subtotal cholecystectomy for "difficult gallbladders": systematic review and meta-analysis. *JAMA Surgery* 2015; 150: 159-168.

Laparoscopic Cholecystectomy in Acute Cholecystitis

Laparoscopic cholecystectomy has emerged as the treatment of choice for acute cholecystitis. *Surgery should ideally be performed in the first week of the onset of an attack.* The outcome of early cholecystectomy is comparable to late cholecystectomy (surgery beyond six weeks) in terms of conversion to open cholecystectomy, morbidity and mortality. The reported advantages of early surgery are: shortened hospital stay, reduced hospital cost and early return to work.

Diagnosis of acute cholecystitis

A. Local signs of inflammation
   1. Murphy's sign
   2. Right upper abdomen mass/pain/tenderness
B. Systemic signs of inflammation
   1. Fever
   2. Elevated CRP
   3. Leukocytosis
C. Imaging findings: characteristic of acute cholecystitis

Suspected diagnosis: One each of A and B
Definite diagnosis: One each of A and B + C
Acute hepatitis, other acute abdominal diseases, and chronic cholecystitis should be excluded
Source: Yokoe M, Takada T, Strasberg SM. New diagnostic criteria and severity assessment of acute cholecystitis in revised Tokyo guidelines. *Journal of Hepatobiliary Pancreatic Sciences* 2012; 19: 578–585.

Severity assessment criteria for acute cholecystitis

Grade I: (Mild) – Acute cholecystitis in a healthy patient with no organ dysfunction and only mild inflammatory changes in the gallbladder

Grade II: (Moderate) – Acute cholecystitis is accompanied by any one of the following conditions:
1. Elevated WBC count ($>18,000/mm^3$)
2. Palpable tender mass in the right upper abdominal quadrant
3. Duration of complaints >72 hours.
4. Marked local inflammation (gangrenous cholecystitis, pericholecystic abscess, hepatic abscess, biliary peritonitis, emphysematous cholecystitis)

Grade III: (Severe) Acute cholecystitis is accompanied by dysfunctions in any one of the following organs/systems:
1. Cardiovascular dysfunction: Hypotension requiring treatment with dopamine ≥ 5 µg/kg per minute, or any dose of dobutamine
2. Neurological dysfunction: Decreased level of consciousness
3. Respiratory dysfunction: PaO_2/FiO_2 ratio <300
4. Renal dysfunction: Oliguria, creatinine >2.0 mg/dl
5. Hepatic dysfunction: PT-INR >1.5
6. Haematological dysfunction: Platelet count $<100,000/mm^3$

Source: Yokoe M, Takada T, Strasberg SM. New diagnostic criteria and severity assessment of acute cholecystitis in revised Tokyo guidelines. *Journal of Hepatobiliary Pancreatic Sciences* 2012; 19: 578–585.

DOI: 10.1201/9781003174547-9

Treatment guidelines for acute cholecystitis (Modified Tokyo 2018 guidelines)

Grade I: (Mild)
Early laparoscopic cholecystectomy.

Grade II: (Moderate)

- Early laparoscopic cholecystectomy in a fit patient if *advanced laparoscopic techniques are available*.
- Initial conservative treatment followed by delayed/elective laparoscopic cholecystectomy in patients with associated comorbidities.
- Early / urgent percutaneous cholecystostomy if no response to conservative treatment.

Grade III: (Severe)

- Initial supportive care to reverse organ dysfunction followed by early laparoscopic cholecystectomy by experienced surgeon/advanced center.
- Urgent/early percutaneous cholecystostomy if no response to supportive care, followed by elective cholecystectomy after recovery from acute illness.

Source: Okamoto K, Suzuki K, Takada T et al. Tokyo Guidelines 2018: flowchart for the management of acute cholecystitis. *Journal of Hepatobiliary Pancreatic Sciences* 2018; 25: 55–72.

Operative considerations in acute cholecystitis

- Port placement should be flexible, depending upon the findings after initial evaluation. Extra port may be required to retract for better visualization.
- Retract structures with care.
- Identify landmarks – cystic lymph node and Rouviere's sulcus and follow the principle of 'clearing and review'.
- Use suction irrigation liberally to keep the operative field clean.
- Use blunt dissection, preferably suction cannula to dissect & display structures.
- Dissect in the subserosal plane (between peritoneum and GB wall).
- Keep a gauze piece in the operative field, especially where stone spill is anticipated, to limit indiscriminate spillage of stones and also to use as tamponade for ooze from inflammatory tissues.
- Gallbladder bed ooze or bleed: Use gauze pressure tamponade for 5–7 minutes. Bipolar or spray coagulation may be used. If significant oozing persists, pack the gallbladder fossa with hemostatic agents like Surgicel (oxidized cellulose) or Gelfoam (gelatin sponge) and watch for 10–15 minutes.
- Extract all spilled stones and give copious irrigation and wash in the gallbladder fossa and the Morrison's pouch.
- Extract gallbladder and stones in an endobag.
- Place subhepatic drain selectively before closure.

Anticipated problems and solutions in acute cholecystitis

Dissection	Findings	Anticipated problems	Solutions
Gallbladder	Edematous, distended and tense.	Difficulty in grasping and retracting	Decompress the GB. Use strong tooth grasper
	Gangrenous, friable.	Difficulty in handling. Risk of stone spill	Evacuate the contents and stones. Use serrated grasper for holding GB.
	Impacted stone in the Hartmann's pouch	Difficulty in grasping and dissection. Identification of anatomy difficult	Disimpact the stone into the GB or incise the GB and extract the stone and proceed to dissection
CVS display	Inflamed and obscure hepatocystic triangle	Injury to bile duct and hepatic artery	Identify landmarks and stay in the safe zone Dissect in the subserosal plane Use blunt dissection
	Dense inflammatory adhesions, anatomy not defined	Bilio-vascular injury	Subtotal cholecystectomy
Gallbladder bed	Severe, inflammation, localized perforation Gangrene of the wall	Bleeding from the liver bed	Dissect on the GB wall Do not breach the cystic plate Subtotal cholecystectomy

Issues during difficult laparoscopic cholecystectomy

When it is difficult to establish CVS:

In acute on chronic cholecystitis or gangrenous gallbladder, it may be difficult to establish CVS for the safe clipping of the cystic duct and artery. The following strategies can be adopted in such situations:

- Identify the cystic artery on the gallbladder and lateral to the cystic lymph node, clip and divide. This may facilitate the dissection of the CVS.
- Proceed with subtotal cholecystectomy or cholecystostomy if anatomy is difficult to define.

When to convert:

Conversion at the appropriate time can prevent vascular or bile duct injury. The decision of conversion is directly influenced by the technical skills and experience of the surgeon. In situations like unclear anatomy, lack of progress during dissection and limited experience, conversion should be planned and an open cholecystectomy should be undertaken.

ACUTE CHOLECYSTITIS: OPERATIVE FINDINGS

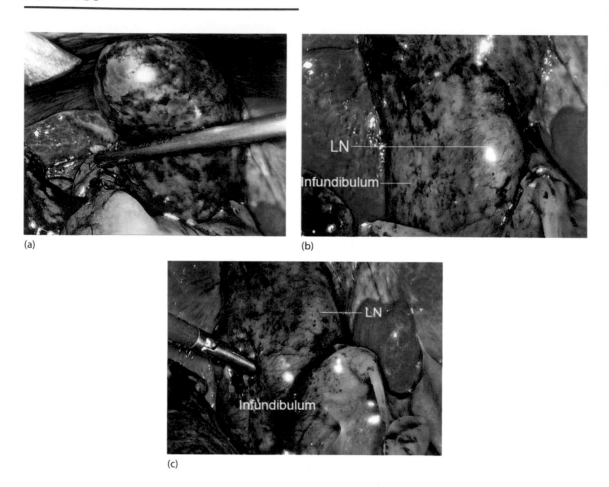

(a)

(b)

(c)

Figure 9.1 **(a)** Gallbladder wall showing patchy gangrene. **(b)** Note the enlarged cystic lymph node. **(c)** The hepatocystic triangle is obliterated with inflamed oedematous tissue.

OPERATIVE STEPS

Gangrenous Cholecystitis: Video v11

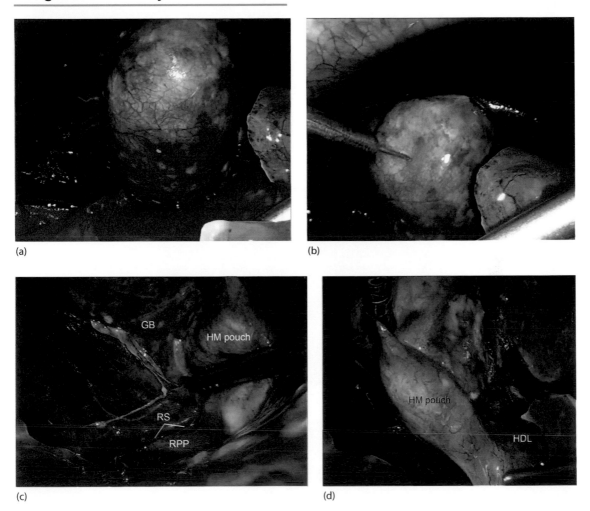

(a)

(b)

(c)

(d)

Figure 9.2 **(a)** Inflamed, distended gallbladder **(b)** decompressed by an aspiration needle. **(c)** The Hartman's pouch is lifted up and the stone disimpacted. Note Rouviere's sulcus and the right portal pedicle. **(d)** Anterior view of the hepatocystic triangle. *(Continued)*

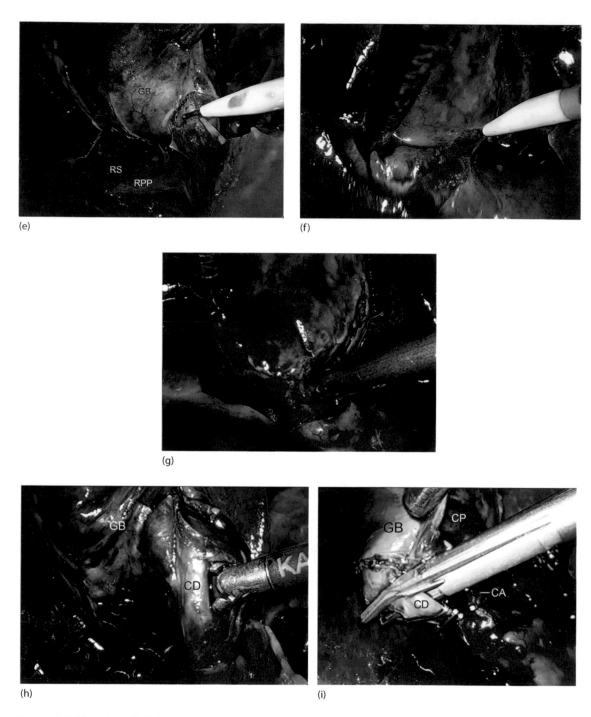

Figure 9.2 (Continued) **(e)**. Posterior peritoneum is incised with electrocautery. **(f)** Anterior peritoneum is incised close to the gallbladder wall and the hepatocystic triangle is dissected. **(g)**. Dissection of the hepatocystic triangle is carried out using a blunt instrument (suction cannula). **(h, i)** The cystic duct and cystic artery are isolated and clipped.

(Continued)

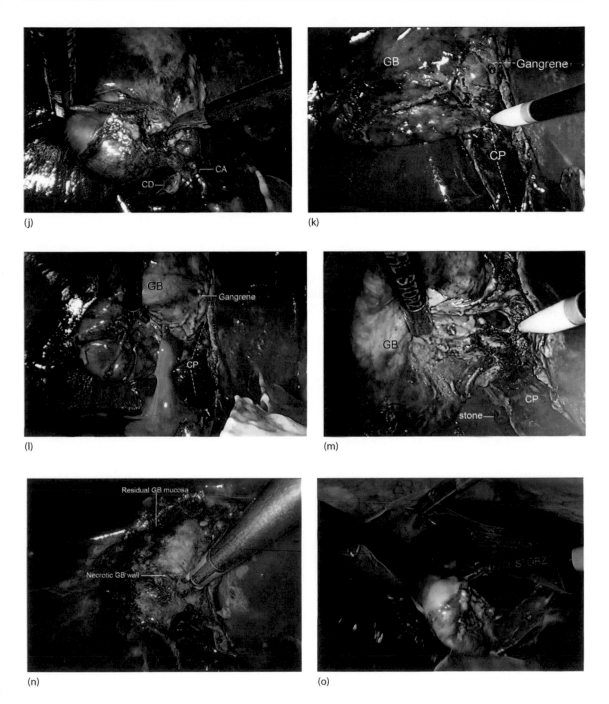

Figure 9.2 (Continued) (j) The cystic duct is divided and the cystic artery is divided close to the gallbladder. (k) The gallbladder is lifted from its bed in the subserosal plane. Note the gangrenous patch visible on the posterior wall. (l) Spillage of pus from the gangrenous gallbladder. (m) The gallbladder is lifted off its bed, partly leaving behind the adherent necrotic wall. Note the dropped stone. (n). The gallbladder bed is cauterized for hemostasis. The adherent necrotic gallbladder wall and mucosa is ablated with cautery coagulation. (o) The gallbladder and the dropped stone(s) are retrieved in an endobag (indigenously prepared polythene bag).

ACUTE CHOLECYSTITIS

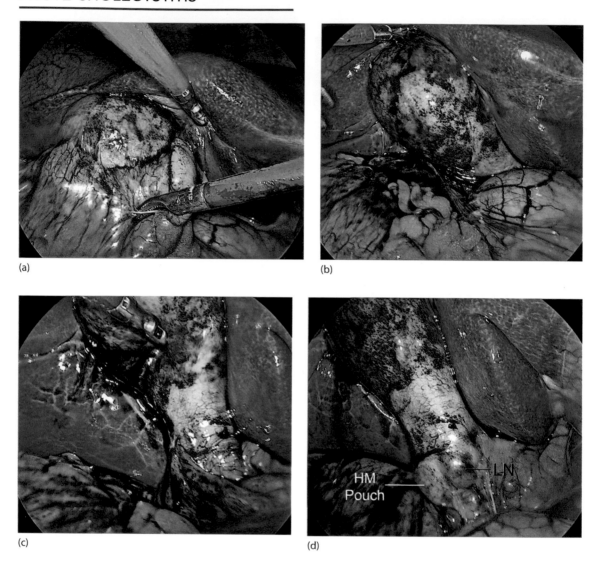

Figure 9.3 **(a)** Omentum adherent to inflamed gallbladder. **(b)** Gallbladder after adhesiolysis. **(c)** Posterior view of the gallbladder. Rouviere's sulcus is absent. **(d)** Anterior view. Cystic lymph node is the only visible landmark. *(Continued)*

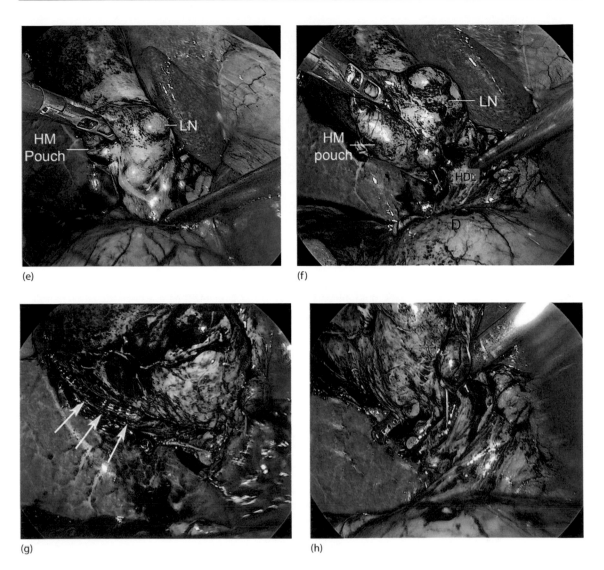

(e)

(f)

(g)

(h)

Figure 9.3 (Continued) **(e)** Dissection started remaining close to the lymph node, using a blunt instrument (suction cannula). **(f)** Blunt dissection of the hepatocystic triangle in progress. **(g)** Incised posterior peritoneum (arrows). A plane is created by mobilizing the gallbladder in the subserosal plane. **(h)** Anterior dissection: The gallbladder is dissected in the subserosal plane. A window is created between the gallbladder and the cystic plate. Note the instrument across the gallbladder in the dissected window.

(Continued)

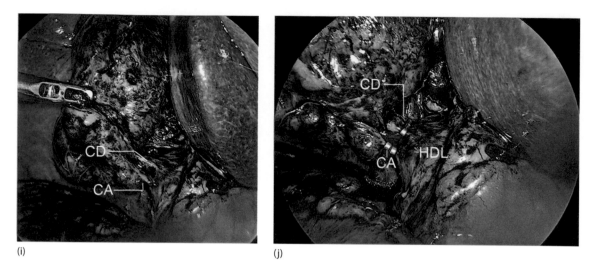

Figure 9.3 (Continued) **(i)** The cystic duct and artery can be appreciated as the hepatocystic triangle is being dissected. **(j)** CVS is achieved. The isolated cystic duct and artery are clipped and divided.

ACUTE ON CHRONIC CHOLECYSTITIS – CVS NOT ACHIEVABLE

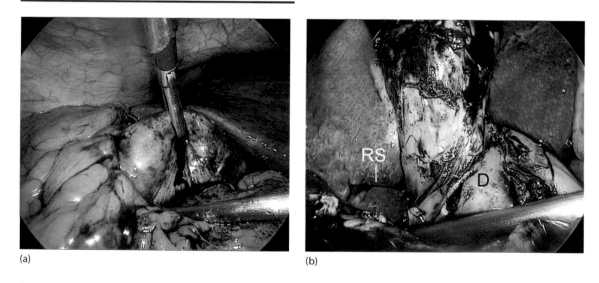

Figure 9.4 **(a)** Inflamed and thick-walled gallbladder is firmly wrapped in omentum. It is held with a strong tooth grasper and remaining close to the serosal surface adhesions are brought down. **(b)** After complete adhesiolysis operative landmarks are identified. Note Rouviere's sulcus and the corresponding portal pedicle.

(Continued)

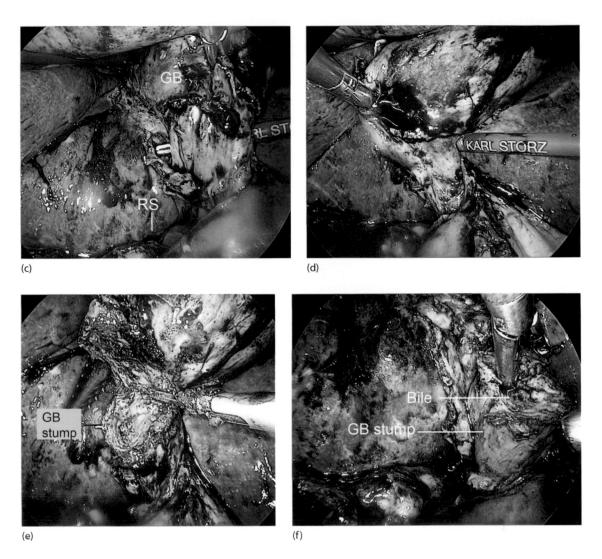

(c)

(d)

(e)

(f)

Figure 9.4 (Continued) **(c)** Posterior peritoneum above the level of Rouviere's sulcus is incised and dissection is carried out. Attempt to dissect the hepatocystic triangle is unsuccessful due to dense fibrosis. Hence a tunnel is created between the gallbladder neck and liver bed. **(d)** Anterior view of the tunnel. **(e)** Using an ultrasonic coagulator, the gallbladder is transected at the neck. **(f)** Note the grossly thick-walled stump. Bile staining in the stump indicates cystic duct opening.   (*Continued*)

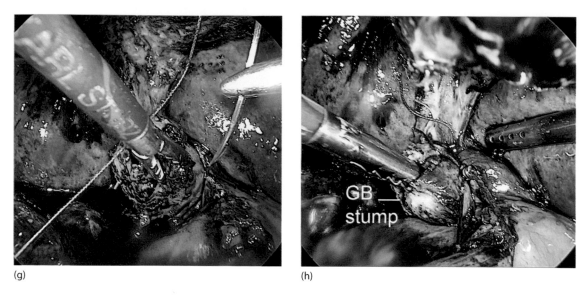

(g)   (h)

Figure 9.4 (Continued) **(g, h)** The gallbladder stump is transfixed with 0–2 Vicryl suture, reinforced with a catgut endoloop.

Laparoscopic cholecystectomy in acute cholecystitis can be challenging. Dissection is carried out close to the gallbladder in the subserosal plane. Suction cannula is used as a blunt dissector and also to keep the operating field clean. These are some of the key steps to achieve CVS. Alternative techniques, such as subtotal cholecystectomy, may prove useful when CVS is not definable due to various reasons.

10

Laparoscopic Cholecystectomy in Special Situations

OVERHANGING LIVER SEGMENTS

Hypertrophy and/or congenital lobulation of the liver segments can obscure the gallbladder and make it inaccessible for dissection.

Issues and strategy

- Hartman's pouch and the hepatocystic triangle are difficult to access due to overhanging liver segments.

- Extra ports may be required for the retraction of the overhanging liver.
- Division of peritoneum, proper retraction and dissection close to the gallbladder help in achieving CVS.
- Alternatively, mobilization of gallbladder body followed by antegrade dissection remaining close to the gallbladder can provide access to structures in hepatocystic triangle.

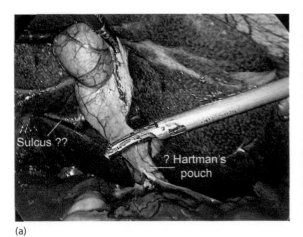
(a)

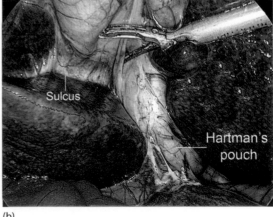
(b)

Figure 10.1 **(a)** Distal body and the Hartman's pouch are obscured by the overhanging liver segments. A sulcus lateral to the gallbladder simulating Rouviere's sulcus can be seen. **(b)** With adhesiolysis and fundal traction, the obscured segment of the gallbladder along with the Hartman's pouch becomes apparent. The sulcus is a result of lobulations of the liver segments. The hepatocystic triangle is not approachable as it is hidden underneath the overhanging liver. Hence, dissection is started proximally with division of the posterior peritoneum near the body. *(Continued)*

DOI: 10.1201/9781003174547-10

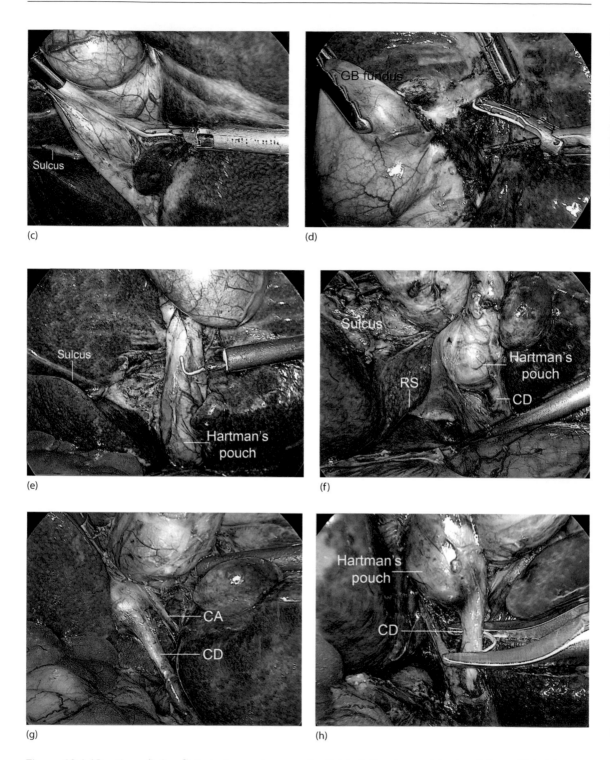

Figure 10.1 (Continued) **(c, d)** Anterior peritoneum is divided. Fundus and body of the gallbladder are mobilized. **(e)** After complete mobilization from its bed, the gallbladder is retracted cranially. **(f)** This exposes the posterior aspect of the hepatocystic triangle and also the Rouviere's sulcus. **(g)** Anterior view of the dissected cystic duct and artery. **(h)** Cystic duct, posterior view.

STONE IMPACTED IN THE RETROCHOLEDOCHAL CYSTIC DUCT: Video v13

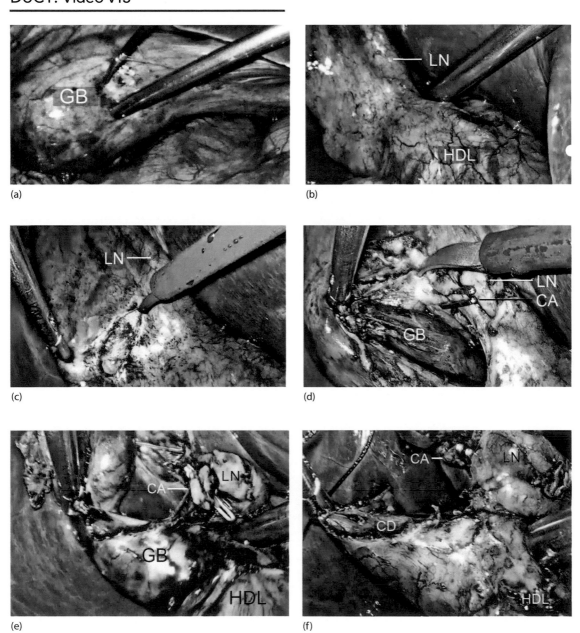

(a)

(b)

(c)

(d)

(e)

(f)

Figure 10.2 **(a)** Distended gallbladder (mucocele) is decompressed with suction cannula. **(b)** Note the wide cystic duct, and the indistinct junction beween infundibulum and hepatoduodenal ligament. **(c, d)** Anterior peritoneum is incised and the gallbladder is mobilized in the subserosal plane. The cystic artery is dissected, clipped and divided. **(e)** Mobilized gallbladder. **(f)** The infundibulum is suture ligated and the cystic duct is transected. The impacted stone can be felt through the hepatoduodenal ligament. Attempt to manouevre the stone out of the cystic duct is unsuccessful. *(Continued)*

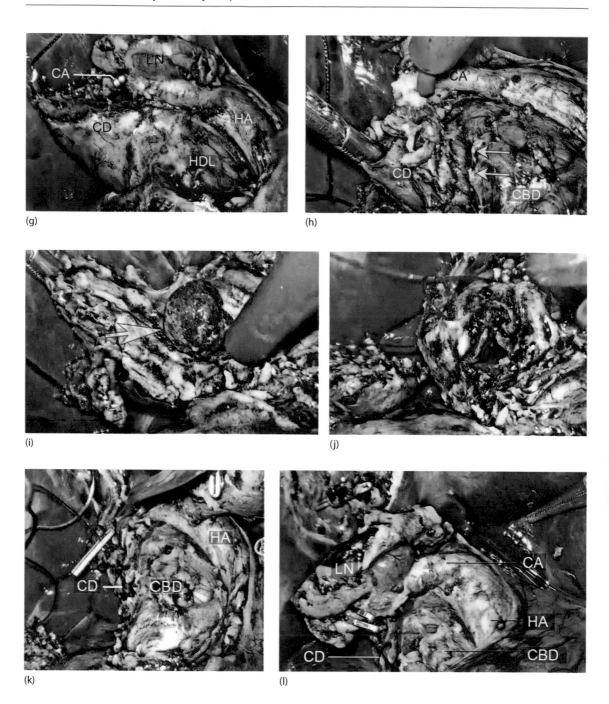

Figure 10.2 (Continued) **(g).** The cystic duct stump is mobilized further by dividing the peritoneum and dissecting the hepatoduodenal ligament. **(h)** Note the dissected margin of the cystic duct (arrows) as it courses behind the common bile duct. **(i)** Incision is given over the stone (arrow) and it is delivered. **(j)** The cystic duct stump is closed by continuous 3-0 PDS suture. **(k)** Sutured cystic duct stump posterolateral to common bile duct. **(l)** Displayed structures after completion of the cholecystectomy. *An impacted stone causing mucocele of the gallbladder must be carefully looked for and retrieved.*

A stone in the cystic duct running posterior to CBD is technically difficult to access and there is a risk of this stone being missed and left behind.

ABERRANT HEPATIC ARTERY:
Video v14

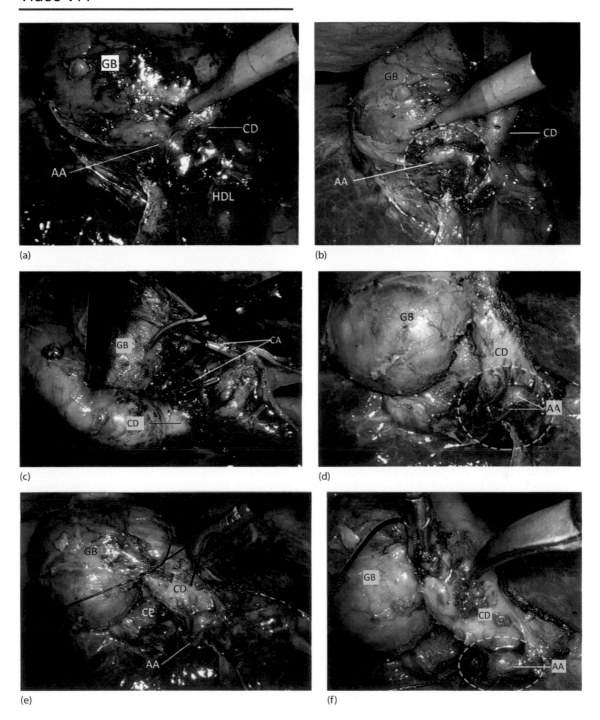

Figure 10.3 **(a)** Impression of an aberrant artery can be seen on the inferolateral aspect of the gallbladder neck. **(b)** The artery (dotted circle) is exposed by dividing the overlying peritoneum with an L hook. **(c)** The hepatocystic triangle is exposed anteriorly. The cystic artery is replaced by two small arterial twigs which are clipped, coagulated and divided. **(d)** The cystic duct appears wide and is merging with the infundibulum. The aberrant artery is seen running across the cystic duct at its base (dotted circle). **(e, f)** The distal part of the gallbladder is mobilized from its bed (cystic plate), encircled with a silk ligature and divided.

(*Continued*)

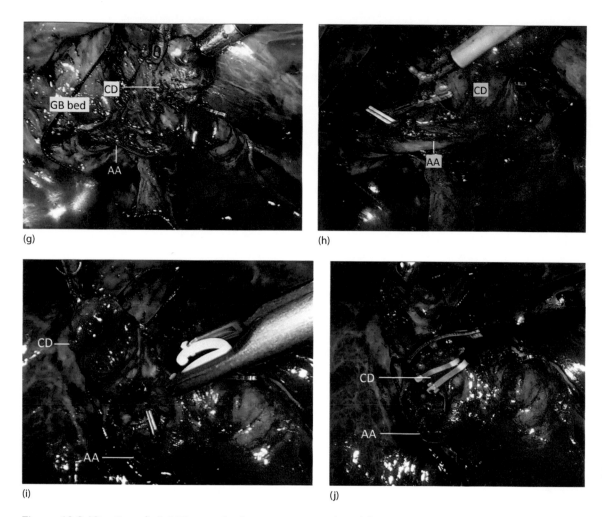

Figure 10.3 (Continued) **(g)** The cystic duct stump is explored for any residual stone or debris. **(h)** It is mobilized further by dissecting it free of the adherent artery. **(i, j)** The cystic stump is defined and clipped and the excess part excised.

An aberrant artery of such calibre is likely to be the right hepatic artery or its segmental division. Hence, care must be taken to identify, dissect and preserve it.

MIRIZZI'S SYNDROME

Mirizzi's syndrome is defined as obstruction of the common bile duct by stone in cystic duct or Hartman's pouch. The obstruction can be due to external compression (Mirizzi type I) or by erosion of the stone into the common bile duct through cholecysto-choledochal fistula (Mirizzi type II-IV). Management of Mirizzi's syndrome includes confirmation of diagnosis by MRCP and a preoperative endoscopic biliary stenting with CBD stone extraction (if present). The hepatocystic triangle is generally obliterated and not amenable to dissection. Subtotal cholecystectomy is the treatment of choice for Mirizzi (type I-III). Traditionally, considered a contraindication for laparoscopic surgery, with increasing familiarity with laparoscopic dissection and suturing, all the steps of open subtotal cholecystectomy can be performed by laparoscopy.

Operative technique

- Adhesions are separated to expose the gallbladder.
- Preliminary dissection is done to assess the hepatocystic triangle and local anatomy.
- Gallbladder is opened near the Hartman's pouch or on the impacted stone. After removing stone(s), the gallbladder is visualized from inside for presence of cholecystocholedochal fistula.
- Mirizzi Type I-III can be managed by laparoscopy and subtotal cholecystectomy.
- Gallbladder is excised, leaving behind approximately one cm cuff adherent to CBD/ around the cholecystocholedochal fistula.

- Gallbladder cuff is closed (choledochoplasty) with a 3.0 PDS suture.
- Alternatively, a T-tube of appropriate size may be kept in the CBD and the vertical (long) limb is brought out through a fresh choledochotomy. Though less desirable, the long limb of the tube can also be brought out through the gallbladder cuff. The latter is associated with higher incidence of postoperative bile leak.
- A subhepatic drain is placed.
- Mirizzi's syndrome type IV which requires a Roux Y hepaticojejunostomy may have to performed by conversion to open surgery.

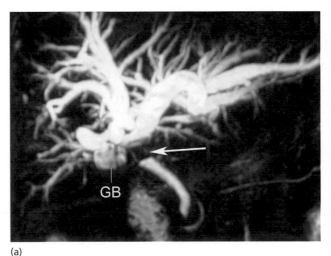

(a)

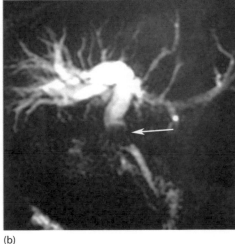

(b)

Figure 10.4 **(a)** MRCP showing a large stone in the mid-CBD with proximal dilatation. **(b)** Stone and 'peg'-shaped deformity of CBD are more apparent in the lateral view. These findings are suggestive of Type II/III Mirizzi's syndrome. *(Continued)*

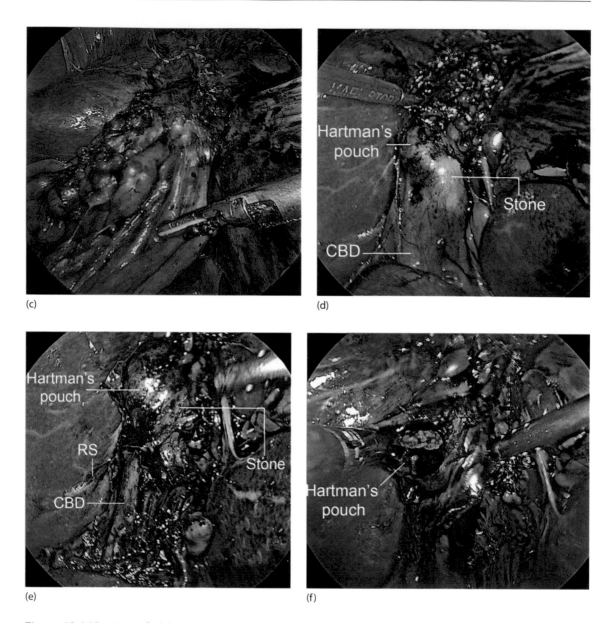

Figure 10.4 (Continued) **(c)** Dense subhepatic adhesions. **(d)** Hartman's pouch, distal undilated CBD and the obstructing stone causing significant mid-CBD bulge are apparent after adhesiolysis. **(e)** Hartman's pouch and the distal CBD are defined. **(f)** The Hartman's pouch is incised and stones are evacuated.

(*Continued*)

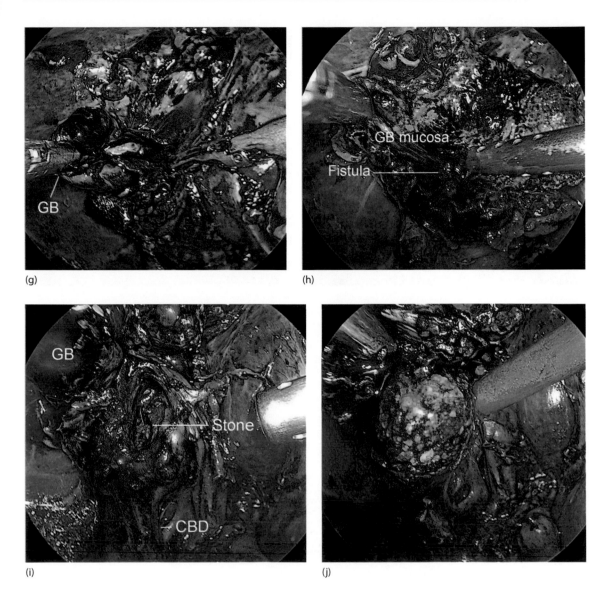

Figure 10.4 (Continued) **(g)**. Fundus of the gallbladder is mobilized and excised. **(h)** The gallbladder is laid open and the cholecystocholedochal fistula is identified. The gallbladder wall is trimmed, leaving behind a cuff of approximately 1 cm around the fistula. **(i)** The mid-CBD bulge is defined and the stone is palpated using grasping forceps. A longitudinal choledochotomy is performed over the stone. **(j)** The stone being delivered out. *(Continued)*

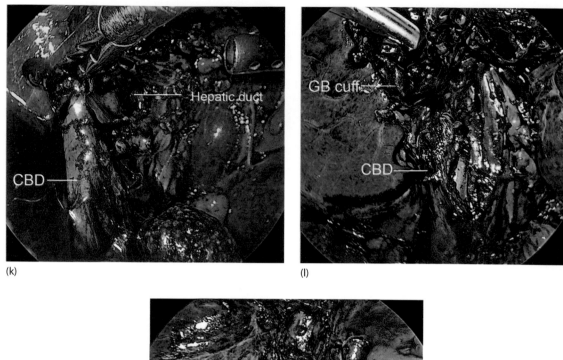

(k)

(l)

(m)

Figure 10.4 (Continued) **(k)** Interior of CBD after the obstructing stone is dislodged. Note the hepatic duct opening at the apex. **(l)** A 14f T-tube is appropriately trimmed. The horizontal limb is placed in the CBD and the vertical limb is brought out through the gallbladder cuff. **(m)** Choledochotomy is closed with an interrupted Vicryl 2-O suture. The gallbladder cuff is approximated around the exiting T-tube. *Alternatively, the vertical limb of the T-tube can be brought out through the choledochotomy with closure of the gallbladder stump and the choledochotomy. T-tube exiting through the GB cuff is associated with a higher incidence of postoperative bile leak and the resultant morbidity.*

CHOLECYSTODUODENAL FISTULA:
Video v15

Cholecystoduodenal fistula (CDF) results from chronic inflammation of the gallbladder and stone erosion into the adjacent duodenum. Laparoscopic cholecystectomy in such a situation is extremely demanding. Traditionally considered an indication for conversion to open cholecystectomy, cholecystoduodenal fistula can be managed by laparoscopy in expert hands. Missed CDF during the release of dense adhesions is a cause for postoperative bile leak, collection and sepsis.

Issues and strategy

- Inflammatory fibrosis and adhesions are real challenges to dissection.

- Dense adhesion between the gallbladder and the duodenum should arouse suspicion of fistula between the two structures.
- The fistula is divided by sharp dissection. Disruption of fistula by blunt dissection results in frayed tissues that is difficult to suture.
- The surgeon must be well conversant in laparoscopic suturing technique.
- Duodenal opening should be closed with interrupted delayed absorbable sutures.
- 'Watertightness' of the closure must be confirmed by an air leak test.
- Conversion to open cholecystectomy must be considered if faced with difficulty at any stage.

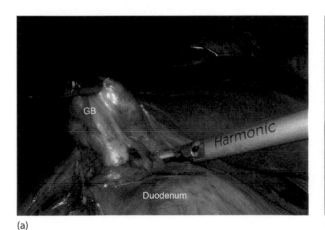

(a)

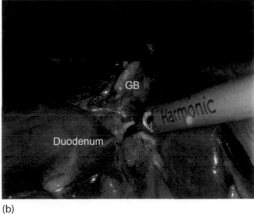

(b)

Figure 10.5 **(a)** Contracted gallbladder and dense subhepatic adhesions. **(b)** Duodenum is densely adherent to the gallbladder. Both blunt and sharp dissection is performed to define the planes.   (*Continued*)

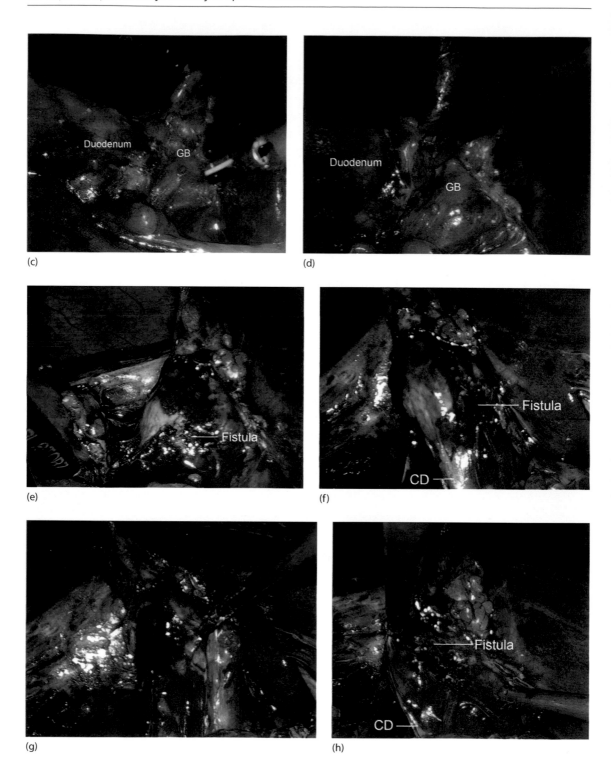

Figure 10.5 (Continued) **(c)** Duodenum appears inseparable from gallbladder, suggesting a fistulous communication between the two. **(d)** The fistulous communication is divided with scissors. **(e)** The opening of the fistula in Hartman's pouch is identified. **(f)** The gallbladder is dissected to identify structures in the hepatocystic triangle. **(g)** Posterior view of the hepatocystic triangle. **(h)** Anterior dissection.

(Continued)

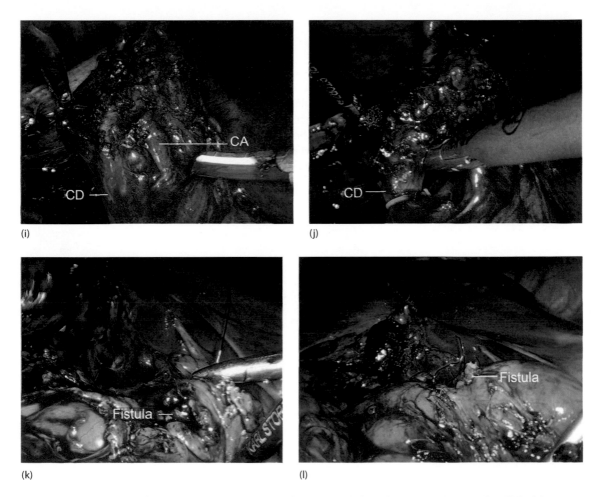

Figure 10.5 (Continued) **(i)** Dissection is carried further to define the cystic duct and gallbladder junction. **(j)** Cystic duct is clipped and divided. **(k)** The duodenal opening is defined and closed with 3-0 PDS interrupted sutures. **(l)** Closed duodenal fistula. Integrity and watertightness of the closure is tested by insufflating stomach and duodenum with air and checking for any leak. A tube drain is placed in the subhepatic space before closure.

RESIDUAL GALLBLADDER: COMPLETION CHOLECYSTECTOMY

Completion cholecystectomy is indicated for a symptomatic patient with stone recurrence in the residual gallbladder. Residual/recurrent stones in the GB stump are usually a consequence of a 'reconstituting type' of subtotal-cholecystectomy performed in a difficult situation, wherein the anatomy is obliterated due to acute or acute on chronic inflammation.

Issues and strategy

- Preoperative MRCP is mandatory to define the road map for the surgeon.
- Altered anatomy, inflammatory fibrosis and adhesions are real challenges to revision surgery.
- A non-existent/obliterated hepatocystic triangle limits the scope of dissection.
- Port placement may require modification to facilitate adhesiolysis and suturing if required.
- Intraoperative ICG cholangiogram may prove helpful in defining anatomy.
- The surgeon should remain prepared to convert to open cholecystectomy at any stage of difficulty.
- Revision surgery must be performed in specialized center by experienced surgeon.

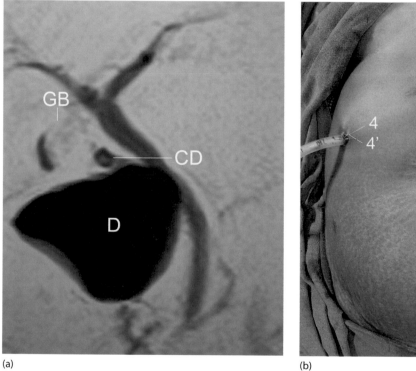 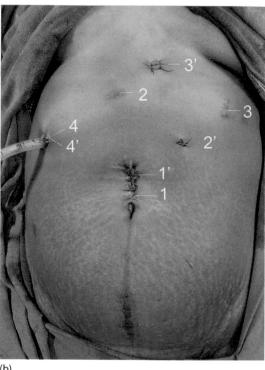

(a) (b)

Figure 10.6 **(a)** MRCP showing stone in the gallbladder stump. **(b)** Port placement: Previous port position 1–4. Current port position 1'–4'. Note that the epigastric port and the midclavicular ports (2', 3') are placed more towards the left to facilitate adhesiolysis and the dissection of the gallbladder.

(Continued)

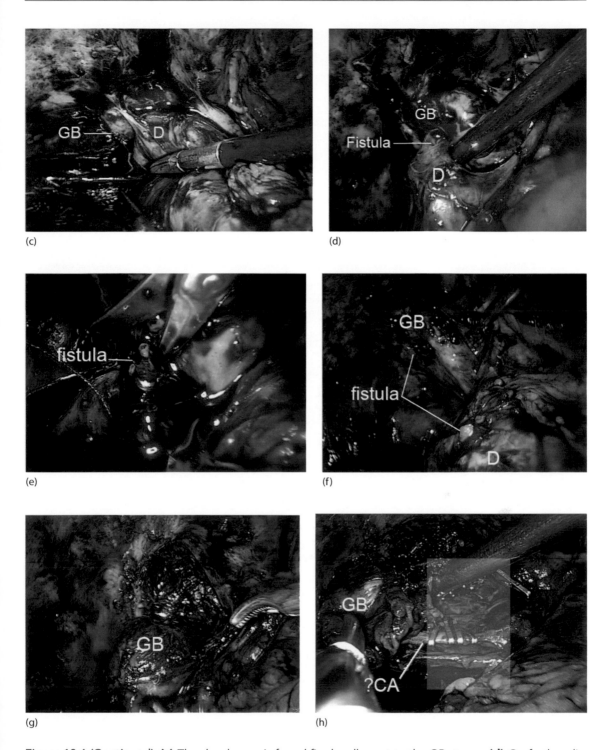

Figure 10.6 (Continued) **(c)** The duodenum is found firmly adherent to the GB stump. **(d)** On further dissection, a fistulous communication between gallbladder and duodenum is found. The fistula is dissected and encircled. **(e, f)** The fistulous tract is ligated, clipped and divided. **(f)** After the division of the fistula, the duodenum is released and mobilized to expose the gallbladder and the subhepatic structures. **(g)** The GB stump is mobilized in an antegrade manner. **(h)** The hepatoduodenal ligament is dissected (shaded area). The cystic artery to the GB stump is clipped and divided. (Continued)

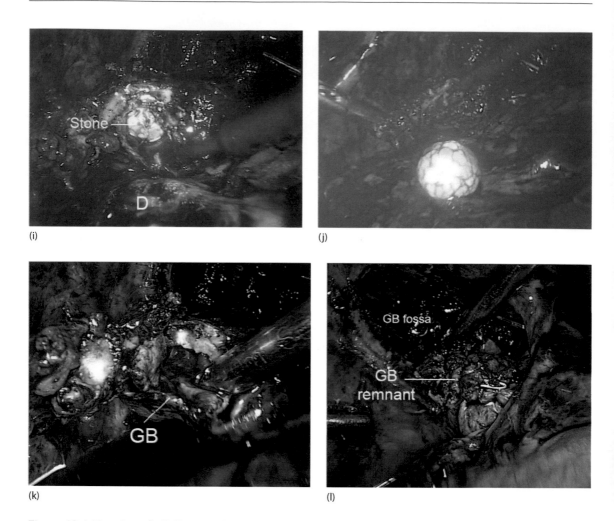

Figure 10.6 (Continued) **(i, j)** Since the hepatocystic triangle is obliterated and the cystic duct is not iden-
tifiable, the GB stump is incised and the stone extracted. **(k)** The excised GB stump is inspected, trimmed
and sutured. **(l)** The approximated GB stump after stone extraction.

Completion cholecystectomy for residual gallbladder is a challenging exercise. Dissection of GB
stump first, coning into the cystic duct, slow and meticulous dissection, help to open up the con-
cealed planes, facilitating the completion cholecystectomy. However, if the dissection appears difficult and unsafe, the GB stump should be incised to extract the stone/s completely. The GB cuff is
approximated after excising the excess margin so as to obliterate the lumen without encroaching
onto the structures in the hepatoduodenal ligament. In redo surgery, the goal is to perform a complete cholecystectomy and thus prevent recurrent symptoms.

11

Laparoscopic Cholecystectomy in Cirrhosis of the Liver and Portal Hypertension

Laparoscopic cholecystectomy is a formidable undertaking in patients with cirrhosis of the liver and portal hypertension. Surgery in patients with Child A & B cirrhosis can be safely performed with great care and caution. In Child C cirrhosis, surgery should be avoided because of operative difficulty as well as the possibility of postoperative liver decompensation.

Issues in cirrhosis and portal hypertension

- The rigid cirrhotic liver prevents adequate retraction and is prone to trauma if excessive traction is applied.
- Operative landmarks and normal anatomy are likely to get distorted due to atrophy, hypertrophy of hepatic segments and regenerating nodules.
- Hypertrophy of the quadrate lobe can obscure the hepatocystic triangle, thereby seriously limiting the access to defining the 'Critical View of Safety'.
- Operative bleeding can get exaggerated due to associated coagulopathy.
- In patients with extrahepatic portal vein obstruction (EHPVO), the difficulty is posed by large collaterals in the hepatoduodenal ligament and the gallbladder wall which is associated with a risk of severe bleeding and also restricts dissection to define the 'Critical View of Safety'.
- Dissection of the posterior wall of the gallbladder from the liver bed can be difficult, with a risk of bleeding due to collaterals.

DOI: 10.1201/9781003174547-11

CIRRHOSIS OF THE LIVER

Case 1

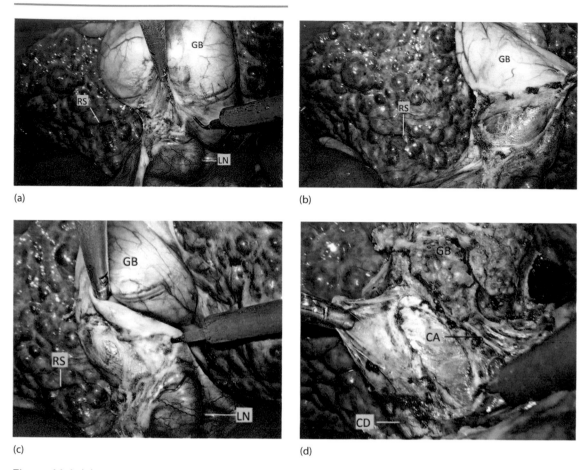

(a)

(b)

(c)

(d)

Figure 11.1 **(a)** Hartman's pouch is gently lifted and Rouviere's sulcus identified. Remaining close to the gallbladder wall, overlying peritoneum is incised. **(b)** Posterior dissection is carried out first. **(c, d)** Anterior dissection on the gallbladder is carried out lateral to the cystic lymph node. *(Continued)*

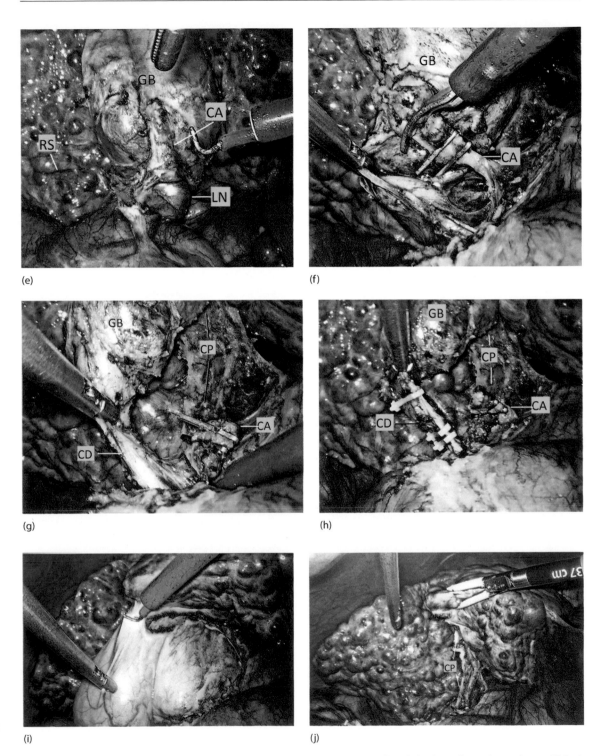

Figure 11.1 (Continued) (e)The cystic artery is isolated, running behind the lymph node to the gallbladder surface. (f) The distal third of the gallbladder is mobilized from the cystic plate. After defining the 'Critical View of Safety', the cystic artery is divided between clips. (g, h) The cystic duct is clipped and divided. (i, j) The gallbladder is mobilized from its bed using an L hook and Ligasure (bipolar cautery). *Even in presence of cirrhosis it may be possible to achieve CVS with careful dissection.*

Case 2

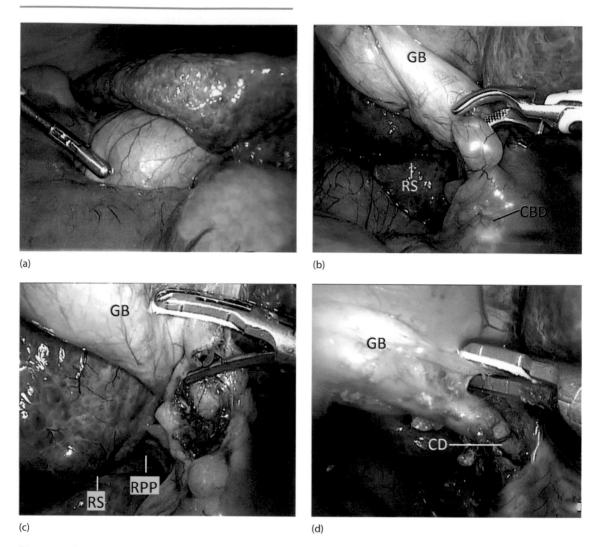

(a)

(b)

(c)

(d)

Figure 11.2 **(a)** Cirrhotic liver. **(b)** Rouviere's sulcus appears deep due to the hypertrophy of liver segments. The hepatocystic triangle appears unremarkable. **(c)** Posterior dissection is performed first. **(d)** Anterior dissection of hepatocystic triangle is performed next.   (*Continued*)

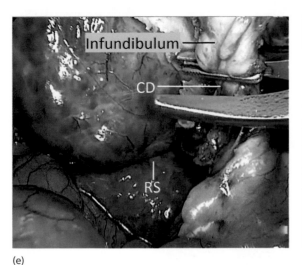

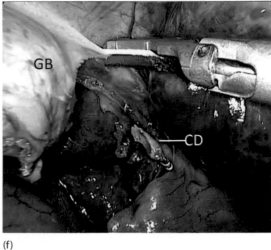

(e)

(f)

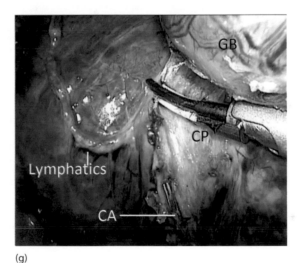

(g)

Figure 11.2 (Continued) **(e, f)** Cystic duct is isolated, clipped and divided after mobilizing the gallbladder from the cystic plate. The cystic artery is, however, not apparent. **(g)** The gallbladder is mobilized and removed from its bed by dividing its mesentery with an ultrasonic coagulator (Harmonic scalpel). Note the dilated lymphatic channels on the liver surface.

Despite cirrhosis, cholecystectomy technically may not be difficult when inflammatory changes and distortion of liver anatomy are minimal.

Case 3

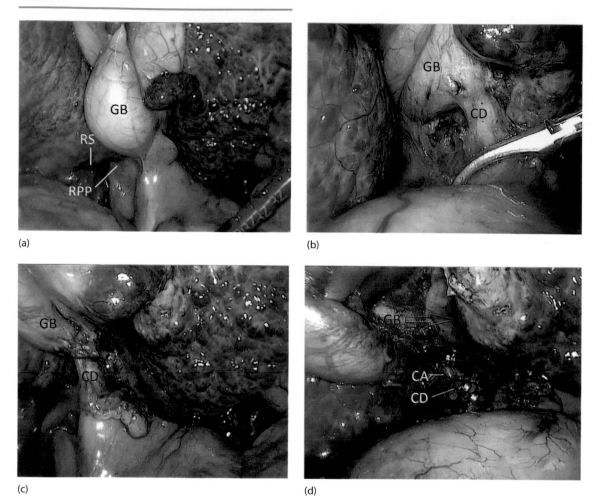

(a)

(b)

(c)

(d)

Figure 11.3 **(a)** The liver appears grossly cirrhotic with distortion of anatomy. **(b)** The posterior dissection is carried out first. **(c, d)** Dissection of the hepatocystic triangle is attempted. Because of the hypertrophy of the quadrate lobe the distal part of the gallbladder appears deeply embedded. This makes obtaining 'Critical View of Safety' difficult and hazardous. Hence, the cystic duct and artery are divided close to the gallbladder. *(Continued)*

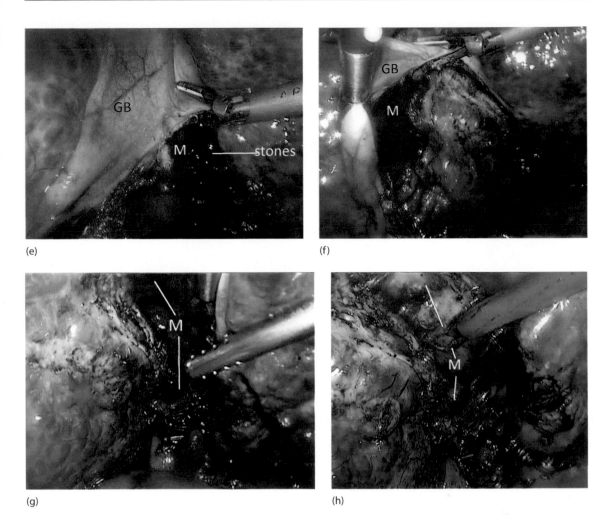

(e)

(f)

(g)

(h)

Figure 11.3 (Continued) **(e, f)** The gallbladder bed appears too deep for safe dissection. Hence, GB is removed, leaving behind the posterior wall adherent to the liver. **(g)** The adherent posterior wall that is left behind. **(h)** The mucosa (M) is cauterized using spatula.

EXTRAHEPATIC PORTAL VEIN OBSTRUCTION (EHPVO): Video v17

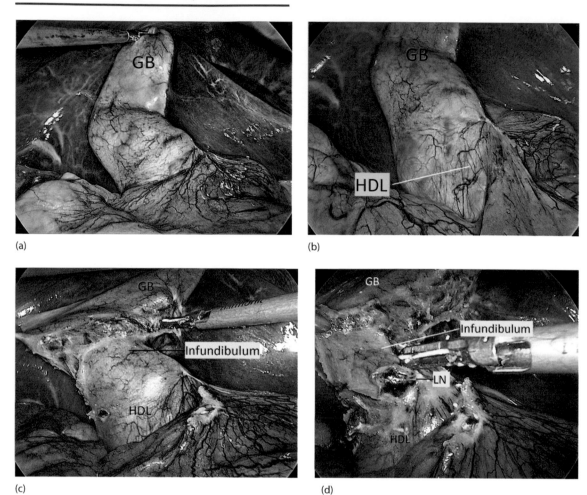

(a)

(b)

(c)

(d)

Figure 11.4 **(a)** Venous collaterals on gall bladder surface. **(b)** Huge dilated, tortuous veins (collaterals) in the hepatocystic triangle and hepatoduodenal ligament obliterating all visible landmarks. **(c)** In the absence of any visible landmark, dissection is started at the gallbladder neck, extending towards the cystic plate. **(d)** The cystic lymph node can be identified after peritoneal incision. Dense collaterals are noticed in the hepatocystic triangle and on the gallbladder surface, making further dissection unsafe. Hence, a decision is taken to go for the fundus-first approach. *(Continued)*

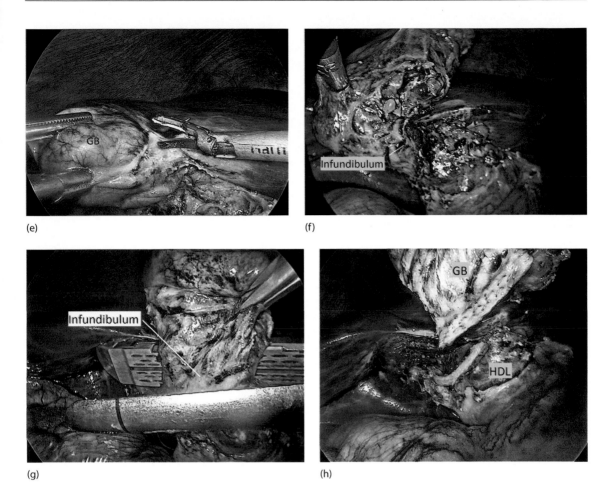

Figure 11.4 (Continued) **(e)** Fundus of the gall bladder is carefully mobilized from its bed using an ultrasonic coagulator (Harmonic scalpel). The plane of dissection is strictly kept between the gall bladder and the cystic plate. **(f)** The gallbladder is mobilized up to the infundibulum. The junction of the infundibulum and the hepatoduodenal ligament is defined. **(g)** In the absence of any definable cystic duct, the gallbladder is divided at the infundibular level with a linear cutter 45 (Ethicon, Johnson and Johnson) that is introduced through the 12mm-epigatric port. **(h)** Note the transected infundibulum is flush to the hepatoduodenal ligament containing huge venous collaterals.

Unlike liver cirrhosis, the presence of dilated, tortuous venous collaterals in EHPVO needs to be handled carefully. In the absence of any definable landmark, particularly the gallbladder and common bile duct junction, it would be prudent to convert to open cholecystectomy. However, the judicious use of an ultrasonic dissector (Harmonic scalpel) for dissection and stapler for transection may help in overcoming the difficulty, as in the present case. Application of stapler where the gallbladder narrows to join the hepatoduodenal ligament should minimize the possibility of retained stone(s) in the remnant.

12

Laparoscopic Cholecystectomy for Malpositioned Gallbladder

Gallbladder malposition has been classified as either medioposition or sinistroposition. A gallbladder in medioposition is displaced medially to the base of segment IV, but is located to the right of the ligamentum teres. In sinistroposition or left-sided gallbladder, the gall bladder is placed to the left of the falciform ligament.

MEDIOPOSITION GALLBLADDER (MIDLINE GALLBLADDER)

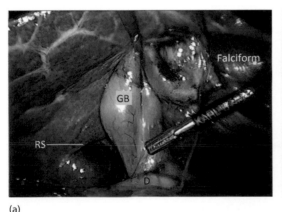

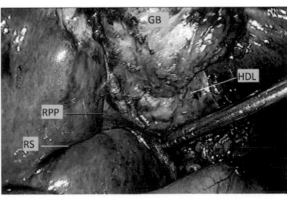

(a) (b)

Figure 12.1 **(a)** The gallbladder is seen attached to segment IV of the liver. The fatty envelope of the gallbladder is merging with the falciform ligament. **(b)** Note the anatomical landmarks in relation to the gallbladder - Rouviere's sulcus, the right portal pedicle and the hepatoduodenal ligament.

(Continued)

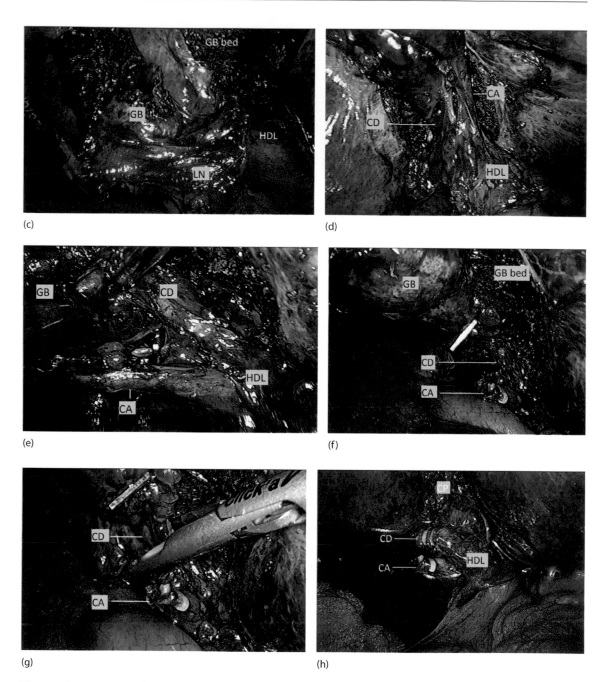

Figure 12.1 (Continued) **(c)** The gallbladder is mobilized by the fundus-first approach till its junction with the hepatoduodenal ligament. The GB is then retracted laterally and dissection proceeds in the routine manner. **(d)** The cystic duct and artery (posterior view) are identified and defined. **(e)** The cystic artery and the duct after isolation (anterior view). **(f)** The cystic artery is clipped and divided. **(g)** The cystic duct is clipped. **(h)** Stumps of the cystic duct and artery after removal of the gallbladder. *(Continued)*

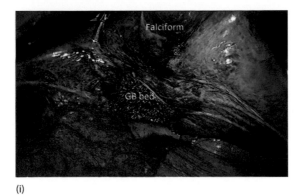

(i)

Figure 12.1 (Continued) (i) The location of the gallbladder, i.e., its midline disposition, can be well appreciated after its removal.

LEFT-SIDED GALLBLADDER

There are three recognized varieties of left-sided gallbladder (LSGB):

1. LSGB associated with situs inversus.
2. True LSGB without situs inversus.
3. Gallbladder located to the left of an anomalous right-sided ligamentum teres.

A true LSGB is located at the base of segment III, to the left of ligamentum teres as well as to the left of the middle hepatic vein. In this variant, the cystic duct may join to the left or right of the common bile duct, or even join the left hepatic duct directly. The cystic artery follows an unusually long course, and crosses in front of the CBD from right to left. Additionally, there may be atrophy of segment IV. The presence of LSGB is associated with a significant risk of biliary injury (4–7.5%) and conversion rates of up to 50%.

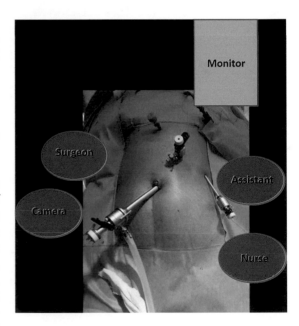

Figure 12.2 Port position and operation theatre arrangement for left-sided gallbladder.

The key steps in a safe cholecystectomy in a left-sided gallbladder are:

- Modify port position (Fig 12.2) and use an additional port for retraction if required.
- Hitch the falciform ligament to the anterior abdominal wall by a suture.
- The classical posterior dissection may need to be modified.
- Dissect by a fundus-first/combined approach, remaining close to the gallbladder.
- ICG cholangiography is recommended if anatomy is unclear.
- Cystic duct is to be divided as the last step after completely mobilizing the gallbladder.

SITUS INVERSUS: Video v18

Laparoscopic cholecystectomy in patients with situs inversus is a challenging proposition in view of changed anatomical disposition. The inversion merits a "mirror image" orientation of the ports and monitor and also that the surgeon stands on the right side of the patient. The ergonomics for a right-hand surgeon is poor and uncomfortable. The epigastric port remains the dissection port but, due to crossing of the surgeon's hands, a lower than usual midclavicular port positioning is ergonomically better and avoids clashing of working instruments.

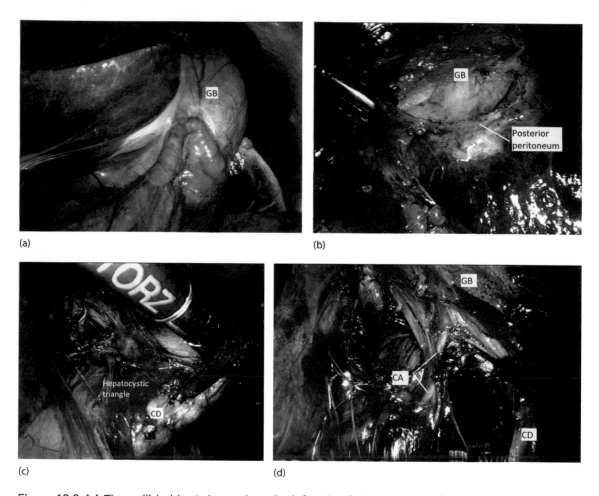

(a) (b)

(c) (d)

Figure 12.3 **(a)** The gallbladder is located on the left side of the abdomen. **(b)** Dissection is begun by incising the posterior peritoneum. **(c)** Hartman's pouch is retracted superiorly towards left to expose the anterior aspect of the hepatocystic triangle. **(d)** The hepatocystic triangle is carefully dissected to expose the cystic artery and the duct.

(*Continued*)

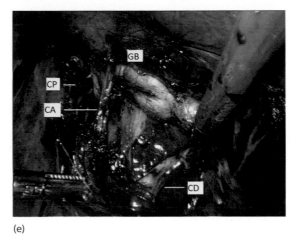

(e)

Figure 12.3 (Continued) **(e)** The hepatocystic triangle is cleared and the distal part of the gallbladder is dissected off the cystic plate to achieve the 'Critical View of Safety'. Note the displayed cystic duct and artery. The cystic artery and duct are clipped and divided and GB removed from the liver bed.

TRUE LEFT-SIDED GALLBLADDER: Video v19

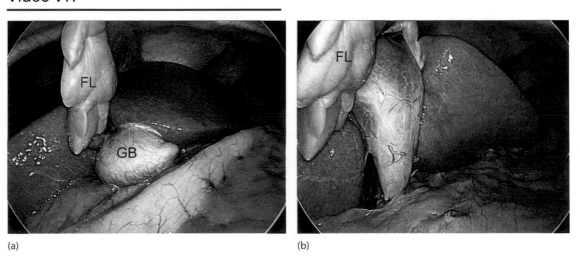

(a)   (b)

Figure 12.4 **(a)** Fundus of the gallbladder is seen on the left side of the falciform ligament. **(b)** The gallbladder is held at fundus and lifted cranially.   (*Continued*)

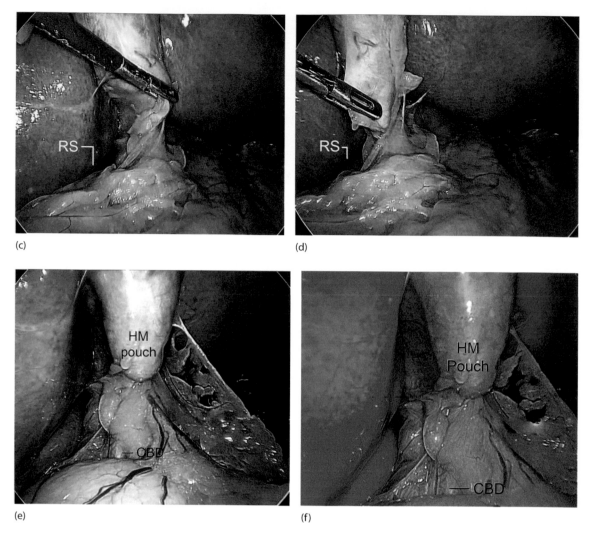

Figure 12.4 (Continued) **(c)** Posterior and **(d)** anterior aspect of the gallbladder. Rouviere's sulcus is seen postero-inferior to the gallbladder. **(e, f)** Before starting dissection, the ICG cholangiogram is performed to assess anatomy. The common bile duct can be appreciated, covered as it is by fat and superior to the duodenum. *(Continued)*

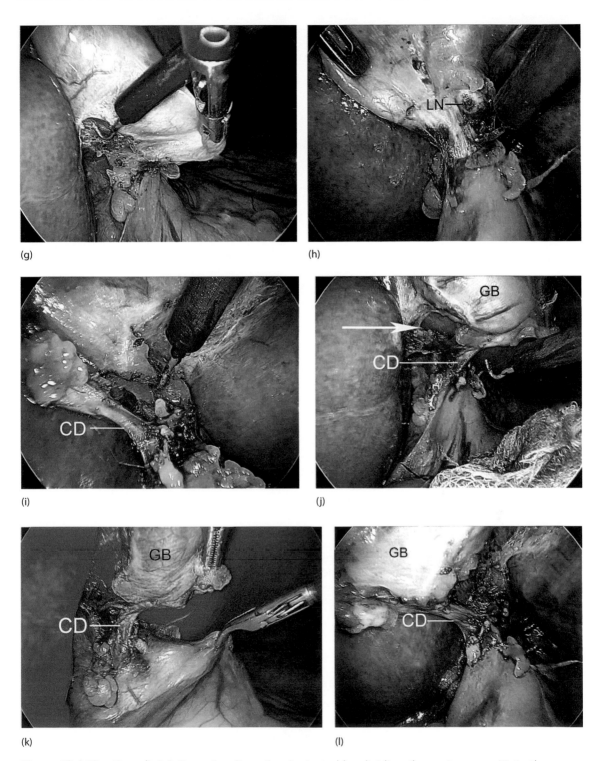

Figure 12.4 (Continued) **(g)** Posterior dissection is started by dividing the peritoneum. Note the crossing of the dissecting instruments. **(h)** Anteriorly, the peritoneum is divided in an attempt to dissect the hepatocystic triangle. Note the cystic lymph node. **(i)** Anterior dissection of the hepatocystic triangle is in progress. **(j)** Window (arrow) created by dissection of the hepatocystic triangle. **(k)** Cystic duct identified and defined during dissection is confirmed by the ICG study. **(l)** Gallbladder is dissected off the cystic plate and CVS is obtained. The cystic duct is isolated, but no separate cystic artery is Identified.

(Continued)

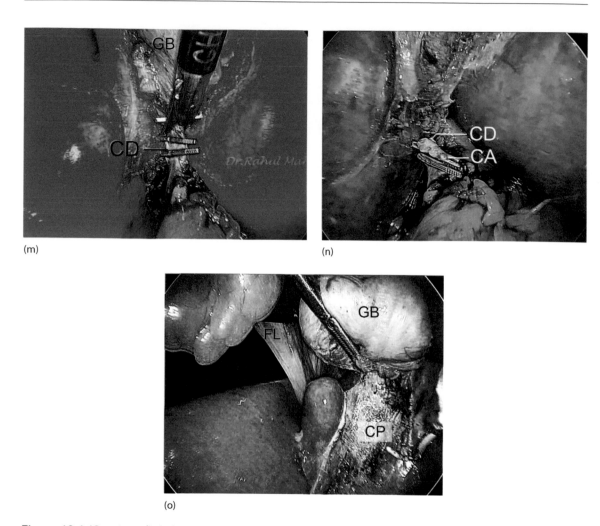

(m)

(n)

(o)

Figure 12.4 (Continued) **(m)** Cystic duct is clipped and divided after confirmation with the ICG study. **(n)** The divided end confirms the presence of both cystic duct and artery inside the clip. **(o)** Gallbladder is dissected off the cystic plate. Note the gallbladder fossa is located medial to the falciform ligament. *This case represents a true left-sided gallbladder associated with atrophy of segment IV. Technically, the dissection requires reorientation. Port placement is modified because of the anatomical necessity. But all other standard steps of surgery, i.e., division of peritoneum, dissection of hepatocystic triangle and obtaining CVS can be performed in the routine manner with relative ease. The minor inconvenience that occurs during dissection is because of the left displacement of gallbladder, which may necessitate the crossing of instruments.*

The gallbladder, when not in its normal location, requires proper judgment and diligence during dissection. The established landmarks are to be identified and located. When it's not possible to demonstrate CVS, a careful antegrade (fundus-first) approach should be adopted. The cystic duct and artery should be carefully defined and divided. The use of cholangiography (ICG) is a useful adjunct, especially in these clinical situations.

13

Intraoperative Cholangiography for the Extrahepatic Biliary Anatomy

Delineation of extrahepatic biliary anatomy during laparoscopic cholecystectomy is required in the following situations: Suspected CBD stone, unclear anatomy and suspicion of bile duct injury. Intraoperative cholangiography (IOC) and fluorescent cholangiography (FC) are the two accepted techniques for this purpose. Several retrospective studies and surveys have shown an association of use of IOC with decreased incidence of bile duct injury and also detection of intraoperative injuries in about 85% of cases when suspected.

INTRAOPERATIVE CHOLANGIOGRAPHY

Intraoperative cholangiogram[1] has been recommended routinely for the detection of bile duct stone/s and delineation of biliary anatomy as a road map for dissection during cholecystectomy. The technique entails dissection of the cystic duct, the placement of a proximal ligation or clip towards the gallbladder, cannulation of the cystic duct, injection of the radio opaque dye, fluoroscopy and imaging.

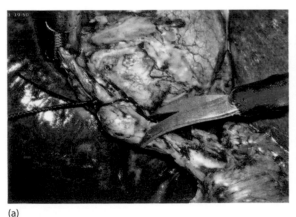
(a)

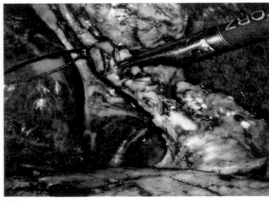
(b)

Figure 13.1 **(a)** After dissection of the cystic duct, ligature is placed proximally (towards the GB) and ductotomy is made on the cystic duct. **(b)** Ductotomy is being probed with a 'right angle' clamp.

(Continued)

DOI: 10.1201/9781003174547-13

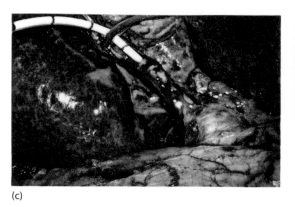

(c)

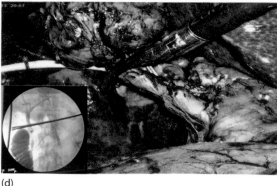

(d)

Figure 13.1 (Continued) **(c)** Cystic duct is cannulated with a 5F ureteric catheter. **(d)** Catheter is secured and cholangiogram performed. *Inset* – Cholangiogram delineating the CHD, right and left hepatic ducts and the CBD with no filling defect. Dye is seen in the duodenum.

Limitations of IOC

a. Operation theatre facility: high-resolution fluoroscopy equipment and expertise are required to conduct an IOC, which may not be available in all institutions (especially in developing countries).
b. It leads to additional operating time and cost.
c. IOC cannot be performed where the cystic duct is blocked.
d. Incorrect interpretation of the biliary anatomy on cholangiograms is seen in 57% of IOC and is a serious limitation.
e. Attempts at performing IOC in a setting of unclear anatomy may lead to a bile duct injury.

FLUORESCENT CHOLANGIOGRAPHY

Fluorescent cholangiography[2] is a novel technique of the intraoperative identification of biliary anatomy. FC, by virtue of displaying the extrahepatic biliary anatomy, may facilitate safe dissection and thus avoid injury

a. The method entails the administration of indocyanine green (ICG) intravenously, 0.05 mg/kg, 30 minutes–6 hours prior to cholecystectomy. Fluorescence and imaging are achieved through a dedicated system of near infra-red light detected by a special lens system.

b. FC defines the components of extrahepatic biliary system with good consistency; CD 96.2% (range 71.4–100%), CHD 78.1% (range 33.3–100%), CBD 72% (range 50.0–100%), and CD-CHD junction 86% (range 25.5–100%).
c. Images are obtained in real time and can be repeated during the course of surgery and various stages of dissection, as opposed to conventional IOC.
d. The visualization rates of various structures increase after the dissection of the hepatocystic triangle, especially of the CD and CD-CHD junction.
e. Due to limited penetration of near infra-red light, successful visualization of biliary anatomy is limited in obese patients and in acute cholecystitis with severe local inflammation.

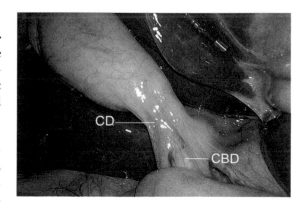

Figure 13.2 Appearance of the biliary system before starting dissection.

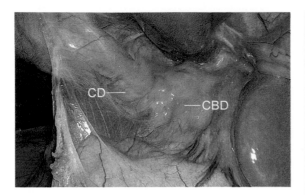

Figure 13.3 Cystic junction and the common bile duct are well delineated.

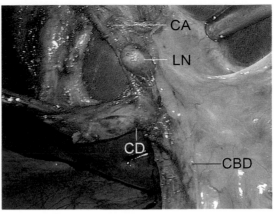

Figure 13.6 The cystic duct appears dilated. Its course, after the delineation of the CVS, can be clearly made out. The cystic duct because of its dilatation can create confusion with CBD.

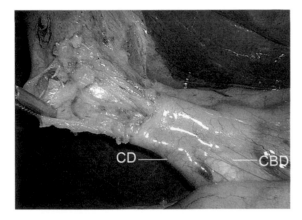

Figure 13.4 Long parallel cystic duct and its relation to CBD.

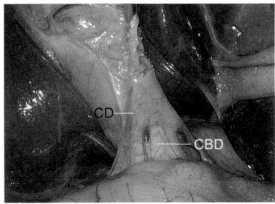

Figure 13.7 Posterior view showing the cystic duct and its proximity to CBD.

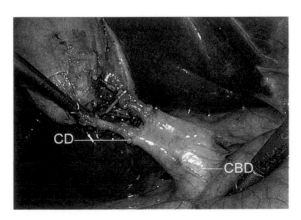

Figure 13.5 Anterior view after dissection of the hepatocystic triangle. The course of the cystic duct is well delineated.

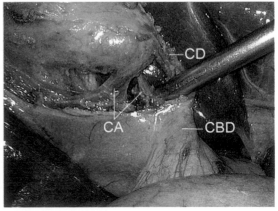

Figure 13.8 Posterior view of CVS showing two cystic arteries and the duct.

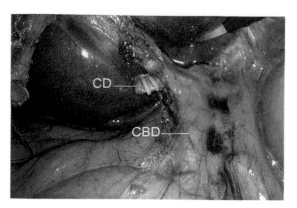

Figure 13.9 Appearance after division of the cystic duct.

Advantages of fluorescent cholangiogram

1. Ease of conducting the study.
2. FC is quicker and cheaper with a very steep learning curve.
3. It provides an opportunity of dynamic real time assessment during all phases of dissection.
4. It is non-invasive, no radiation exposure and useful, even in a blocked cystic duct.
5. No possibility of procedure-related injury to bile duct unlike the conventional IOC.

Recommendations

1. Intraoperative cholangiogram should be performed selectively for the detection of CBD stones, to delineate the extrahepatic biliary anatomy in patients with difficult GB and unclear anatomy or when bile duct injury is suspected.
2. Experienced and trained individuals should undertake the procedure and ensure that complete biliary anatomy is outlined and clearly interpreted.
3. If facilities of FC are available, it should be preferred over IOC to outline the extrahepatic biliary anatomy.
4. Both IOC and FC have limitations in acute cholecystitis and obesity and therefore should be used with caution.

NOTES

1 Ausania F et al. Intraoperative cholangiography in the laparoscopic cholecystectomy era: Why are we still debating? *Surgical Endoscopy* 2012; 26: 1193–1200.
2 Pesce A et al. Utility of fluorescent cholangiography during laparoscopic cholecystectomy: A systematic review. *World Journal of Gastroenterology* 2015; 21: 7877–7883.

14

Troubleshooting during Laparoscopic Cholecystectomy

The common intraoperative issues associated with laparoscopic cholecystectomy (LC) are bleeding, bile leak, bile duct injury and stone spillage. These can cause immediate and long-term morbidity if not managed properly.

BLEEDING: Video v20

Bleeding is a frequent, common but preventable complication during laparoscopic cholecystectomy. Its incidence ranges from 0.04–2.5%, with major uncontrolled bleeding seen in 0.1–1.9% of cases. The common sites of bleed during LC are:

- Gallbladder bed
- Cystic or right hepatic artery
- Port site
- Occasionally, bleeding may arise from major injury to the portal vein or terminal part of the middle hepatic vein in the gallbladder bed.

Major Vascular Injury

The incidence of hepatic artery injury/ligation during LC is in the range 7–13.8%. Isolated RHA clipping or ligation in normal liver and uncomplicated LC may remain unrecognized and asymptomatic. Combined vascular (hepatic artery) and bile duct injury has serious repercussions and impact on the management and outcome of these patients. Portal vein injury is uncommon and is usually a part of a major bilio-vascular injury which needs urgent attention and control. Terminal portion of middle hepatic vein is susceptible to injury during the dissection of the gallbladder bed, especially if the cystic plate is breached. The terminal vein can be as close as <1 mm in 27% of patients and the diameter may vary from 3.2+/−1.1 mm.

Management of bleed during laparoscopic cholecystectomy

The frantic attempt to control bleeding by injudicious cauterization and application of clips is often responsible for the aggravation of bleeding and/or injury to bile duct. We recommend:
- Do not panic.
- Do not cauterize blindly or apply clips indiscriminately.
- Pack the area with gauze and apply pressure.
- Call for help.
- Stop and take stock of the situation
  - o Assess resources, expertise, assistance and vision
  - o Assess severity of bleed
  - o Proceed with laparoscopy or convert to open.

DOI: 10.1201/9781003174547-14

Bleeding from Cystic Artery

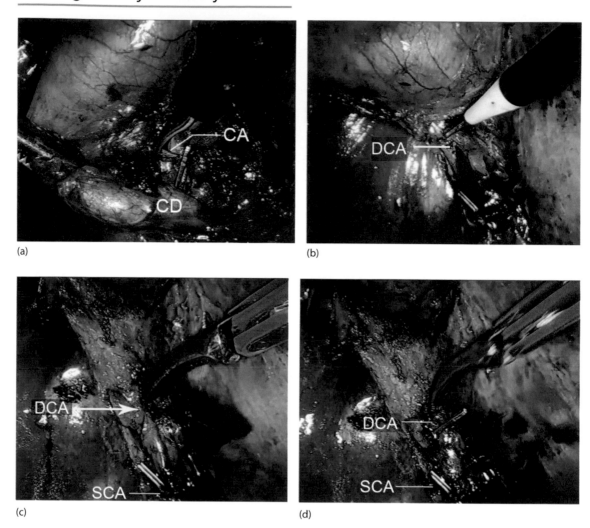

(a)

(b)

(c)

(d)

Figure 14.1 **(a)** Cystic artery is secured in the hepatocystic triangle. **(b)** After dividing the cystic duct and artery, bleeding is encountered during the dissection of the gallbladder from its bed. **(c)** Bleeding appears likely from the deep branch of the cystic artery, the bleeding point is defined and coagulated with bipolar cautery. **(d)** After initial control, a metal clip is applied on it to ensure secure control.

Bleeding from the Gallbladder Bed

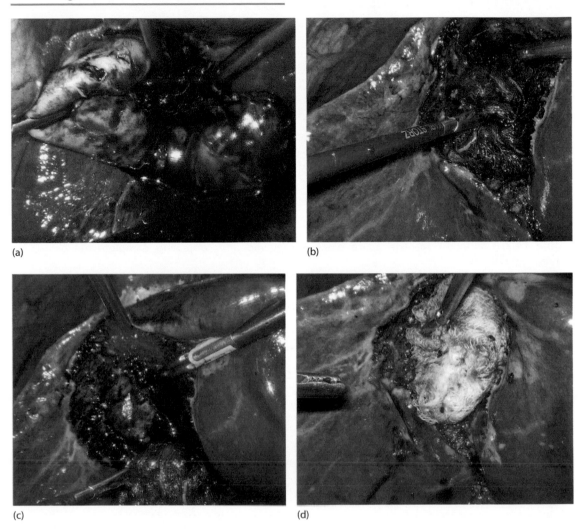

(a)

(b)

(c)

(d)

Figure 14.2 **(a)** Bleeding is encountered during the dissection of the gallbladder from the liver bed. **(b)** The bleeding point is controlled with a gauze piece compression. Dissection and removal of GB is completed. **(c)** The bleeding points are coagulated with bipolar cautery. **(d)** A rolled gauze piece serves well to keep the field clean, helps in retraction of liver and also to maintain pressure during the control of bleeding points by cauterization. (*Continued*)

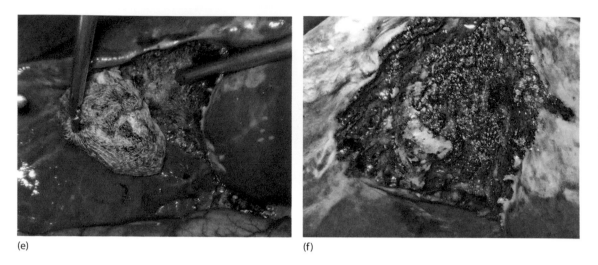

(e)   (f)

Figure 14.2 (Continued) **(e)** The gauze piece is removed after obtaining complete hemostasis. **(f)** Cauterized GB bed.
Venous ooze in the liver bed is best managed with pressure packing, followed by coagulation in spray or bipolar mode.

Bleeding from Hepatic Vein Tributary

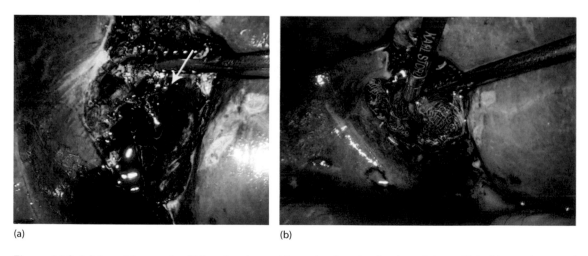

(a)   (b)

Figure 14.3 **(a)** A sudden gush of bleeding (arrow) is noticed as the fundus of the gallbladder is dissected from the liver bed. The bleeding appears venous in origin, and is slow and pulsatile in nature, indicating bleed from the terminal hepatic vein. **(b)** The bleeding point is compressed with a gauze piece and gallbladder dissection from the liver bed is completed.   (Continued)

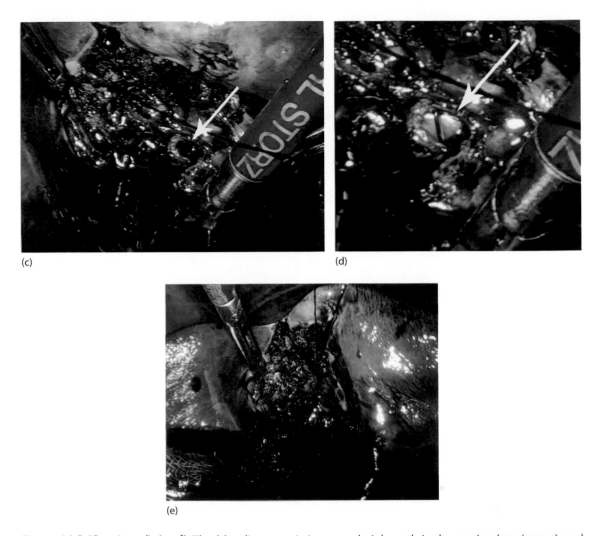

(c)

(d)

(e)

Figure 14.3 (Continued) **(c, d)** The bleeding area is inspected. A breach in the cystic plate (arrow) and a rent in the vein can be identified as the site of bleeding. The venous rent (arrow) is closed with a 3-0 proline suture. **(e)** Surgicel (oxidized cellulose) pack applied to liver bed for further hemostasis.
Bleeding from large hepatic vein tributary is slow and pulsatile in nature. It can be controlled by pressure packing. Significant and persistent bleeding may require suture ligation for control. Occasionally, the bleeding can be massive and catastrophic and may require conversion to open for its control.

BILE LEAK

Bile staining of the operative field during laparoscopic cholecystectomy is not unusual. It is usually a trivial issue resulting from the perforation of the gallbladder during dissection. On rare occasions, it may denote a much more sinister problem such as bile duct injury. Therefore, any bile leak during cholecystectomy, particularly that occurring during dissection of the hepatocystic triangle, should never be ignored. Efforts must be made to identify the source, so that appropriate measures can be taken. The common sources of bile leak are:

- Gallbladder perforation
- Cystic duct rent
- Common hepatic duct/common bile duct injury
- Subvesicle duct

Gallbladder Perforation

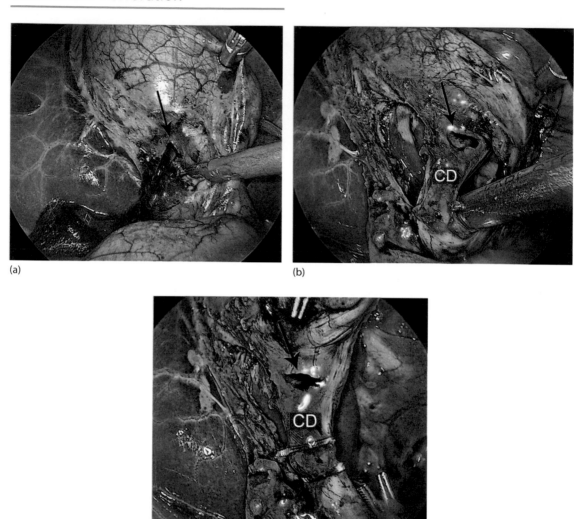

(a)

(b)

(c)

Figure 14.4 **(a)** During the posterior dissection of the gallbladder, an inadvertent thermal injury manifests with a gush of bile (arrow). **(b)** A rent in the infundibulum (the junction of the GB with the cystic duct) is identified on further dissection of the hepatocystic triangle. **(c)** CVS is established and the cystic duct is clearly defined. Two appropriate size clips are placed distal to the rent (arrow) and the cystic duct is divided. *Gallbladder bile is greenish yellow, whereas bile from the bile duct is golden yellow in colour. However, in the absence of infection and patent cystic duct, bile from gallbladder can also appear golden yellow, as in the above case. Such leaks are inconsequential, and require cleaning by suction and irrigation.*

Cystic Duct Injury

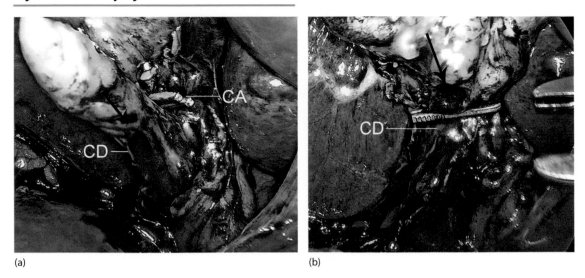

(a)　　　　　　　　　　　　　　　　　　(b)

Figure 14.5 **(a)** Cystic injury during dissection, manifesting as bile spillage. The rent (arrow) in the CD is identified to be close to the common bile duct. **(b)** An appropriate size clip is placed distal to the rent (arrow), taking care to avoid encroachment onto CBD.

Cystic duct injury most commonly occurs while trying to dissect out an adherent cystic artery. A short, dilated cystic duct is more prone to injury during an attempt to encircle it. Once identified, care must be taken to define the site of injury in relation to CBD. An appropriately placed clip often takes care of the bile leak. However, if the rent is too close to CBD, it should be repaired with a fine (3-0 or 4-0) PDS suture and a subhepatic drain should be placed.

Common Bile Duct Injury

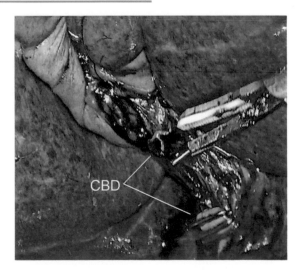

Figure 14.6 The common bile duct has been mistaken as the cystic duct and divided. The transected CBD manifesting as bile soiling of the operative field.

Presence of golden yellow bile, significant size of the divided duct, particularly during dissection in the hepatoduodenal area, should raise the possibility of CBD injury. Confirmation of such an injury requires proper inspection, reviewing the recorded video with an expert and an intraoperative cholangiogram. Once confirmed, the management of the bile duct injury should be undertaken by an experienced surgeon.

Subvesicle Duct

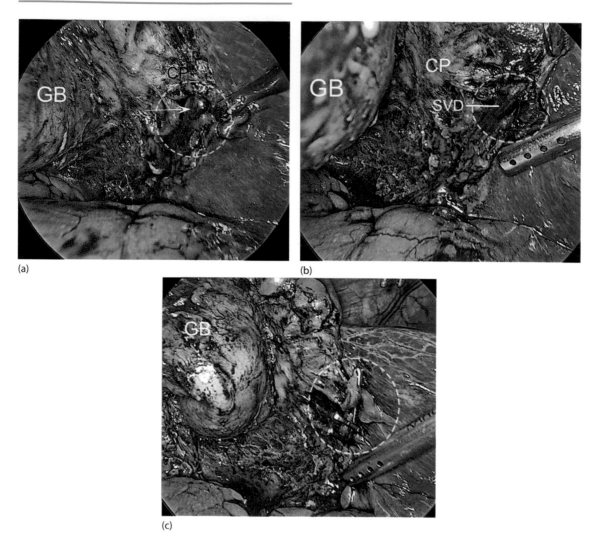

(a)

(b)

(c)

Figure 14.7 (a) Bile staining is noted in the gallbladder bed during its removal. **(b)** The leaking duct is identified as a divided subvesicle duct. The duct is caught with a grasping forceps, slightly lifted and clips are applied at its base. **(c)** The occluded duct with clips.

STONE SPILLAGE

The incidence of gallbladder perforation during laparoscopic cholecystectomy is in the range 10–40% and results in the spillage of bile and stones. The risk of perforation and spillage of stones increases in the elderly and in patients with acute cholecystitis. Stone spillage rate varies from 5 to 30% with a conversion rate for stone retrieval being 5–6%. Residual stones may present with persistent sepsis, intra-abdominal or port-site abscess or persistent cutaneous sinus.

Prevention

1. In the case of thin and inflamed/friable wall and multiple stones, the gallbladder should be decompressed and stones retrieved in a pouch before proceeding to cholecystectomy.

2. In patients with multiple stones and GB perforation during surgery, spread a gauze piece in the subhepatic space to collect the stones and prevent uncontrolled spillage. Entrapped in the gauze piece retrieval of these stones is also easy.

Management of Stone Spillage

1. Ensure that ALL spilled stones are retrieved and placed in an endobag.

2. Search in subhepatic space, in the foramen of Winslow and the subdiaphragmatic space.
3. Use repeated suction and irrigation to remove sludge and small stones. Give thorough saline lavage to remove all infected material.
4. In specific situations, 10 mm suction canula may be used to suck out small spilled stones.
5. Patience and diligence are key to careful picking up all stones.
6. Document stone spill in the operation notes.

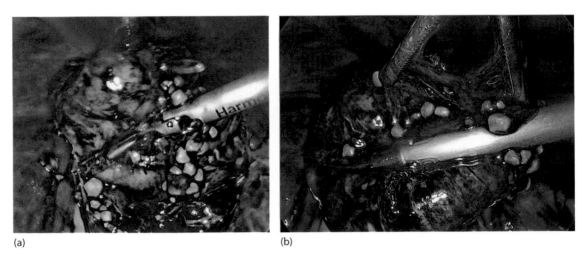

(a) (b)

Figure 14.8 **(a, b)** Stone and sludge spillage during laparoscopic cholecystectomy in a patient with acute gangrenous cholecystitis.

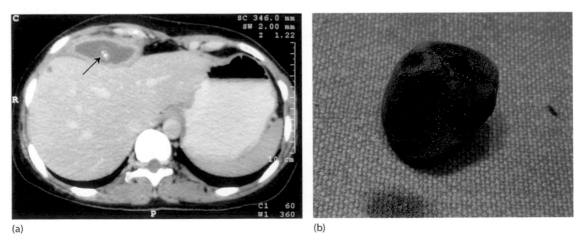

(a) (b)

Figure 14.9 **(a)** Chronic abscess on the antero-superior aspect of liver. Note the radio-opaque calculus (arrow) inside the abscess cavity. **(b)** Recovered gallstone after drainage of the abscess. *The patient had undergone cholecystectomy one year previously and presented with pain and low-grade fever.*

CONVERSION TO OPEN CHOLECYSTECTOMY

Conversion from laparoscopic to open cholecystectomy is a "bail out" option in patients with a difficult cholecystectomy. Conversion rates have decreased over the decades due to improved laparoscopic skills, increasing experience in managing difficult gallbladder and better resolution cameras, including 3D systems and instrumentation. Nevertheless, conversion is more of a judgment call of the surgeon based on the presenting situation and the assessment of resources and expertise. Conversion should NOT be considered a failure of the procedure, but a MATURE judgment call.

Conversion could be an 'elective conversion' as in:

- Anatomy not clearly defined.
- Obliterated hepatocystic triangle with dense adhesions.
- Non-progression of dissection after adequate trial.

Conversion could be a 'forced conversion' as in:

- Bleeding – unable to determine site of bleeding/ uncontrolled bleeding.
- Bile leak from the hilum, anatomy undefined.
- Bile duct injury recognized on the operating table.
- Injury to an adjacent hollow viscera or a large cholecysto-enteric fistula.

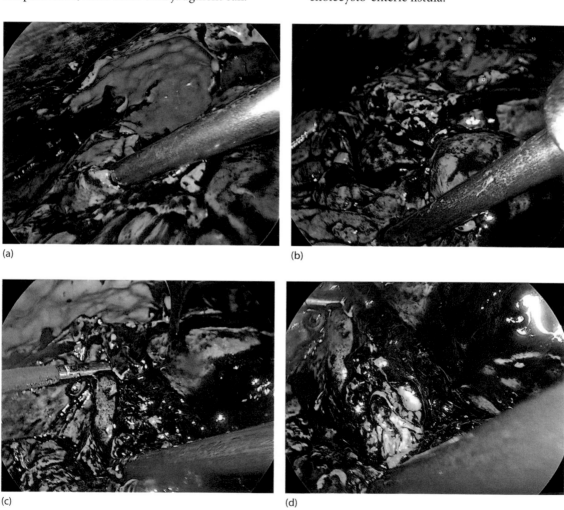

(a) (b)

(c) (d)

Figure 14.10 (a) Acute gangrenous cholecystitis, laparoscopic cholecystectomy in the second week for persistent sepsis. The GB fundus is necrotic. Abscess formation between the liver and the diaphragm in continuity with the necrotic fundus. **(b)** Dense pericholecystic adhesions. **(c)** Adhesiolysis being performed using blunt dissection. **(d)** The hepatocystic triangle is obliterated and cannot be cleared. The colon and the duodenum are densely adherent to the gallbladder. Hence, a decision is taken to convert to open surgery and cholecystectomy.

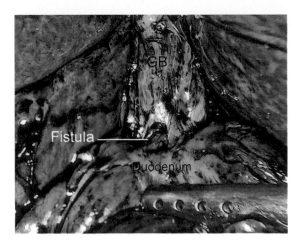

Figure 14.11 Conversion to open cholecystectomy in this patient is decided after encountering a large cholecystoduodenal fistula during laparoscopic dissection.

15

Errors and 'Near Misses' during Laparoscopic Cholecystectomy

Bile duct injury is the most dreaded complication of laparoscopic cholecystectomy, having both immediate as well as long-term implications. The reported incidence of biliary complication is 0.3–1.3% of all cases undergoing laparoscopic cholecystectomy. Various predisposing factors for bile duct injury are listed in Table 15.1. *The infundibular approach to the gallbladder as opposed to the 'Critical View of Safety' approach makes the common bile duct vulnerable to misidentification as the cystic duct. This perception error remains, by far, the most common cause of injury to the bile duct (Fig 15.1).*

Table 15.1 Predisposing factors for bile duct injury

- Altered/obliterated anatomy in the hepatocystic triangle as in acute cholecystitis or long-standing chronic cholecystitis, Mirizzi's syndrome, xanthogranulomatous cholecystitis or portal hypertension.
- Abnormal/aberrant anatomy
- Technical:
  - o Perception error, i.e., misidentification of common bile duct as the cystic duct.
  - o Injudicious use of energy sources and the application of clips to control bleeding.

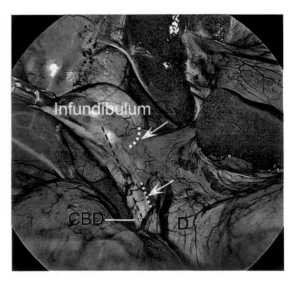

Figure 15.1 Perception error: The hepatocystic triangle is fat-laden, thereby obscuring the anatomy. Common bile duct in alignment with infundibulum (black dotted line) can be mistaken as the cystic duct. This leads to dissection on the medial side of the CBD (dotted straight line and arrow), thereby making the bile duct vulnerable to injury. White dotted curved line (arrow) marks the correct site of dissection. The presence of the duodenum close to the 'apparent cystic duct' should also alert the surgeon about the possible error.

DOI: 10.1201/9781003174547-15

COMMON BILE DUCT INJURY: 'NEAR MISS'

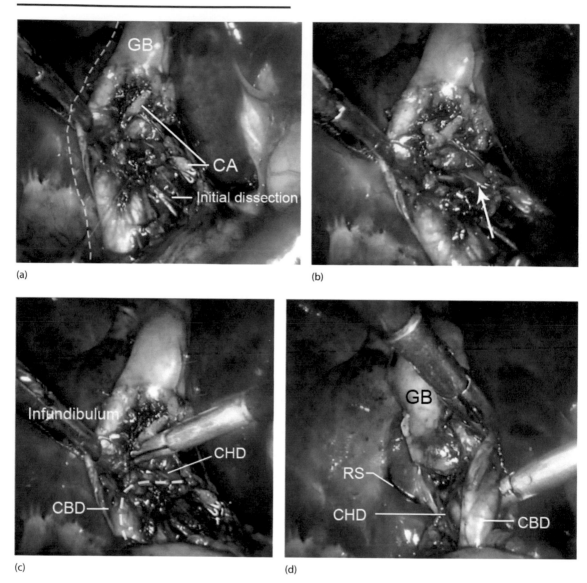

(a)

(b)

(c)

(d)

Figure 15.2 **(a)** The entire segment (dotted line) is presumed as the gallbladder and dissection is started medial to it. The cystic artery is identified, clipped and divided. **(b)** A tubular structure of significant size (arrow) is noticed during dissection. **(c)** On further dissection, it is identified as the CHD coursing from the hilum. The CHD is angulated (dotted line) at its junction with the cystic duct as it continues down as common bile duct. **(d)** Posterior view confirms its position in relation to Rouviere's sulcus.

(Continued)

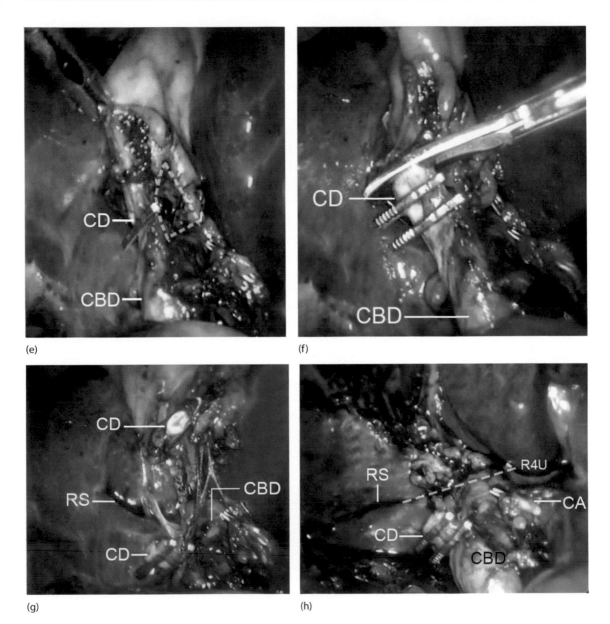

(e)

(f)

(g)

(h)

Figure 15.2 (Continued) **(e)** The hepatocystic triangle (dotted area) is dissected to define the cystic duct. **(f)** The cystic duct, wide in calibre, is clipped and divided. **(g, h)** The CBD is now clearly identified in its normal position after division of the cystic duct. Note the relation of the divided cystic duct with the R4U line.

Summary of events

Initial dissection is carried out medial to the CBD because of a misperception of the extent and boundaries of the gallbladder. The common bile duct is angulated at its junction with the cystic duct due to excessive upward and lateral traction on the infundibulum. The infundibulum, the cystic duct and the common bile duct, lying in a common alignment, appears as one composite structure, i.e., the gallbladder. As the dissection moves upwards, the surgeon's attempt to clear the hepatocystic triangle leads to the identification of the common hepatic duct. At this stage, the mistake is realized, and a major injury to the common duct is averted. The hepatocystic triangle is dissected, cleared and CVS achieved, the cystic duct is identified and the cholecystectomy completed.

Lessons learnt

- Identify landmarks before starting the dissection. In this patient, the initial dissection is below the level of Rouviere's sulcus and the R4U line and close to the duodenum, thereby taking the surgeon medial to the CBD.
- Correct traction is critical – fundus to 10 o'clock position and Hartmann's pouch infero-lateral is required to open up the anterior space for dissection.
- Dissection should remain close to the wall of the gallbladder. Incise the posterior peritoneum and then the anterior peritoneum to facilitate dissection close to the gallbladder and opening up the spaces.
- Clear hepatocystic triangle to define the cystic duct and artery before applying clips or dividing the cystic duct.

MAJOR BILIOVASCULAR INJURY: 'NEAR MISS': Video v21

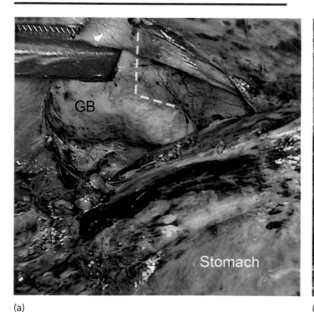
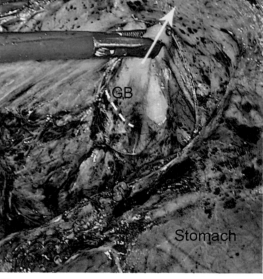

(a)   (b)

Figure 15.3 **(a)** Dense subhepatic adhesions. The contracted gallbladder is seen after adhesiolysis. The area of hepatocystic triangle (dotted lines) is marked. **(b)** Fundus of the gallbladder is retracted medially (arrow). This exposes the postero-lateral aspect of the gallbladder. The dotted line marks the ideal site to start posterior dissection. *(Continued)*

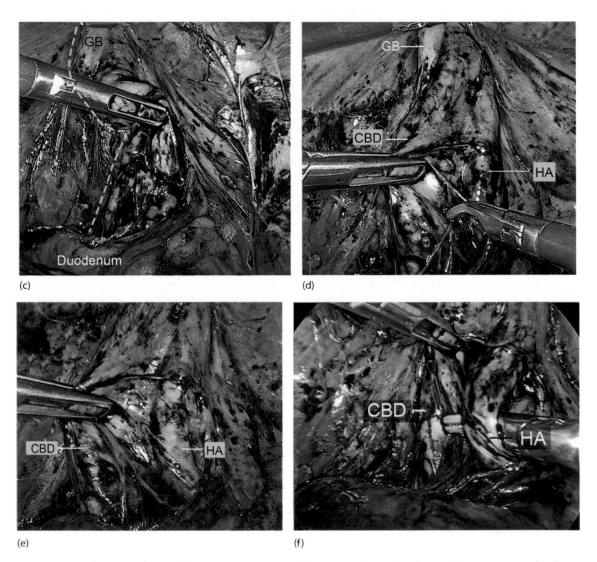

(c)

(d)

(e)

(f)

Figure 15.3 (Continued) **(c)** The stomach and duodenum are brought down, thus exposing the hepatoduodenal ligament. The medially retracted gallbladder along with the dilated CBD is mistaken as single unit – an elongated, distended gallbladder (dotted line) that is extending behind the duodenum. **(d, e)** Dissection commences at the superior border of the duodenum. A large arterial trunk (hepatic artery) on the medial aspect is mistakenly identified as the cystic artery. **(f)** The hepatic artery masquerading as the cystic artery is defined and isolated. (*Continued*)

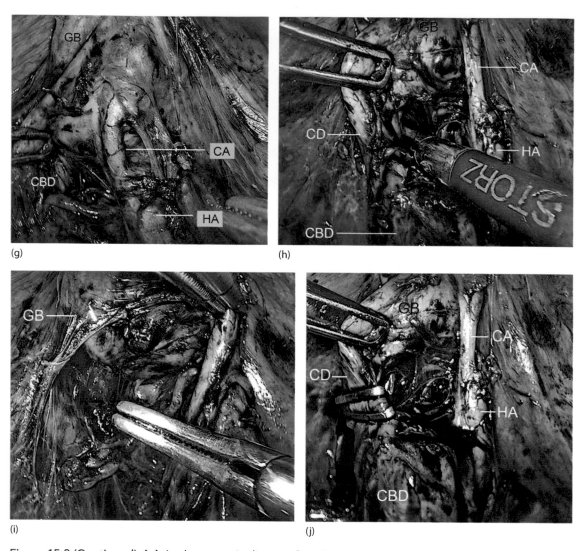

Figure 15.3 (Continued) **(g)** As the artery is dissected up, it is seen coursing towards the hilum after giving off a branch "the cystic artery" supplying the gallbladder. **(h)** Dissection close to the gallbladder wall and lateral to the cystic artery defines the cystic duct. **(i)** Posterior dissection of the gallbladder. **(j)** CVS established; Cystic duct is identified and clipped.

(Continued)

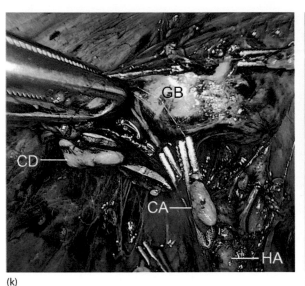
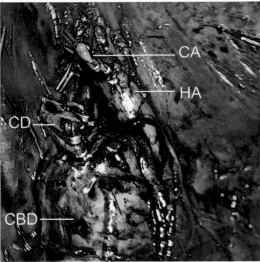

(k)   (l)

Figure 15.3 (Continued) **(k)** The cystic duct and artery are clipped and divided and the gallbladder is removed **(l)** Stumps of the divided cystic duct and artery, the CBD and the hepatic artery, as seen after gallbladder removal.

Summary of events

The subhepatic anatomy is distorted due to extensive inflammatory adhesions, grossly contracted gallbladder and dilated CBD. Medial and upward retraction on the fundus (arrow, Fig. 15.3b) aligns the gallbladder with the CBD to appear as a single entity. This presumed 'elongated gallbladder' can be seen extending behind the duodenum. Dissection is started on the superior border of duodenum. The thick hepatic artery on the medial aspect is misidentified as the cystic artery. It is only when the dissection is carried up to the gallbladder that the proper cystic artery is identified. Subsequent dissection close to the artery identifies the cystic duct. CVS is established and cholecystectomy is thereafter completed in the routine manner.

Lessons learnt

- When the local anatomy is grossly altered, it is important to make a visual assessment of the landmarks before starting dissection.
- Identify the most suitable dissection site. In this case, it is close to the contracted gallbladder as marked (dotted lines) in the pictures (Figure 15.3a, b).
- Retraction of the fundus of the gallbladder in the 10 o'clock direction instead of 12 o'clock, would separate the gallbladder from the CBD.
- The gallbladder, even if elongated in shape, never goes behind the duodenum. Beware if that is the finding!
- Cystic artery should be traced up to the gallbladder before ligation/clipping. This single correct step has averted a major disaster in the present case.

TRANSECTED COMMON BILE DUCT

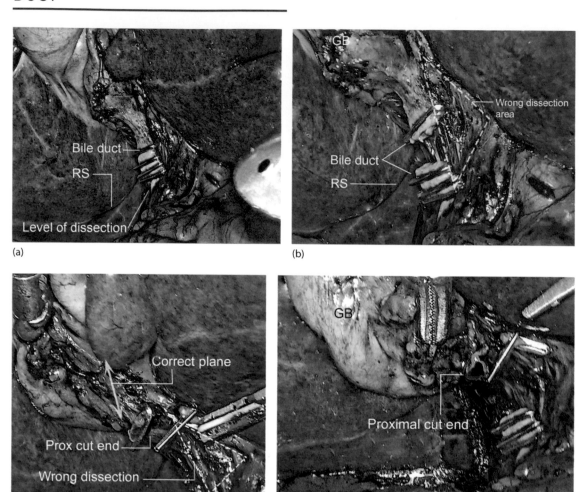

(a)

(b)

(c)

(d)

Figure 15.4 **(a)** Clips are applied on the 'presumed' cystic duct. Note the dissection below the plane of Rouviere's sulcus. The traction on the gallbladder is more towards the 12 o'clock direction. No dissection of the hepatocystic triangle is apparent and CVS not established. **(b)** The "misidentified" cystic duct is divided without establishing CVS. Note that the area of dissection (dotted triangle) is medial to the bile duct. **(c)** As the dissection progresses up and medially (dotted triangle), the proximal transected but clipped CBD becomes apparent. **(d)** The proximal clip gets dislodged with the spillage of golden yellow bile; the wide lumen and direction of the structure confirms the transection of the CBD.   (*Continued*)

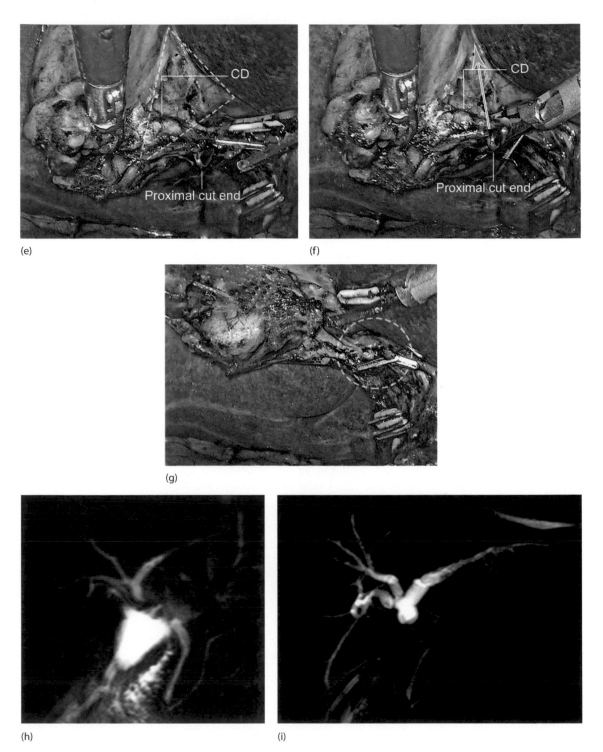

Figure 15.4 (Continued) **(e, f)** As the dissection progresses (with ultrasonic coagulator) from the medial side of the transected duct towards the hepatocystic triangle (dotted triangle and arrow), it further damages the proximal bile duct resulting in excision of a segment of the duct. **(g)** Dissection in the hepatocystic triangle towards the gallbladder bed after the excision of a segment of the common duct (dotted circle). **(h)** MRCP in the postoperative period showing missing bile duct segment and biloma. **(i)** Bismuth Type II stricture in the same patient 5 months later.

Summary of events

The common bile duct is misidentified as the cystic duct because of the retraction of the gallbladder in the wrong direction (10 o'clock) and the dissection plane below Rouviere's sulcus and medial to the bile duct. The duct is clipped and divided without any dissection in the hepatocystic triangle (infundibular technique) and without establishing the CVS. The clues that it could be a transected CBD, i.e., thin-walled, wide tube draining 'golden yellow' bile and coursing towards the hilum, is ignored. In an attempt to remove the gallbladder, the dissection moves from the medial side of the CBD to the hepatocystic triangle, in the process transecting the common duct once more and resulting in the excision of a segment of the common duct.

Lessons learnt

- Adhering to basic principles of laparoscopic cholecystectomy, i.e., the proper retraction of the gallbladder, starting dissection above the plane of Rouviere's sulcus and dividing the structures ONLY after establishing the CVS could have possibly averted the injury.
- A wide tubular structure close to the hilum and draining 'golden yellow' bile should be viewed with the utmost suspicion for a bile duct injury. An intraoperative cholangiogram, if performed at this stage, can identify the bile duct transection.

TRANSECTED COMMON BILE DUCT AND VASCULAR INJURY

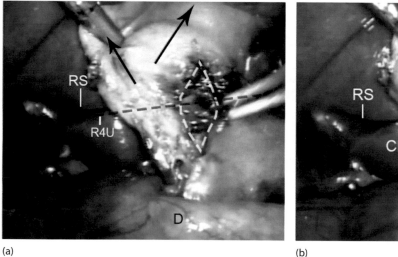
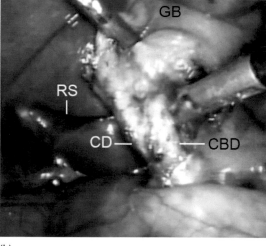

(a) (b)

Figure 15.5 **(a)** Note the direction of retraction of fundus and Hartman's pouch (arrows). The dissection commences medial to presumed infundibulum (dotted area) and below the R4U line (dashed black line). **(b)** The double duct impression of CBD and the cystic duct can be appreciated on close inspection.

(Continued)

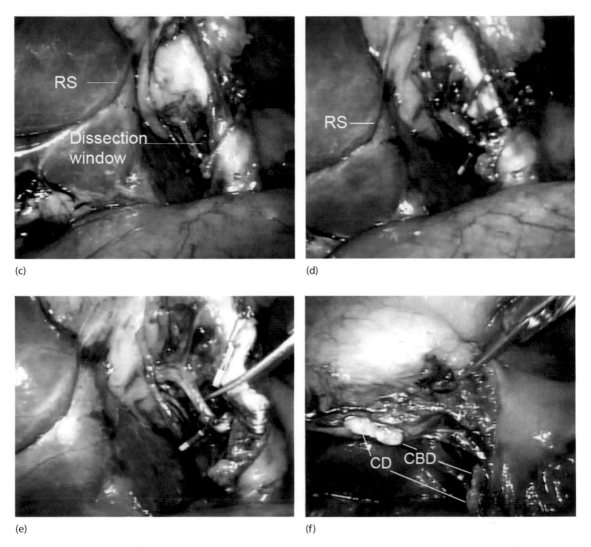

Figure 15.5 (Continued) **(c)** Posterior view – the dissected segment is much below the plane of Rouviere's sulcus and the R4U line. Note the clipped right hepatic artery. **(d)** Clips have also been applied to both the cystic duct and the CBD. **(e)** Division of CBD along with the cystic duct. **(f)** As the gallbladder dissection is carried out bluntly, a longitudinal structure (CHD) is identified from the hilum up to the point of ductal transection. Note the double lumen in the clipped end. *(Continued)*

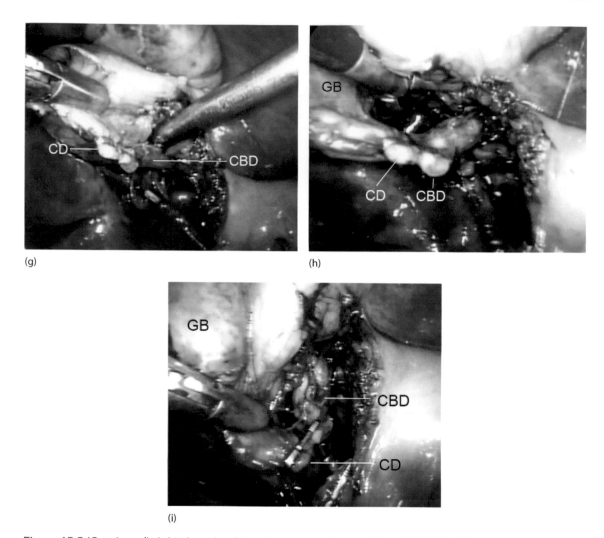

(g)

(h)

(i)

Figure 15.5 (Continued) **(g)** When the dissection proceeds on to the gallbladder, the transected bile duct becomes apparent. **(h)** The transected common duct, along with the cystic duct, is clearly visible as the dissection in the hepatocystic triangle is carried out **(i)** Classic injury of CBD with complete transection. The injury is identified on the table and an end-to-end repair is carried out over a T-tube. *(Continued)*

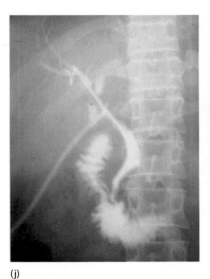
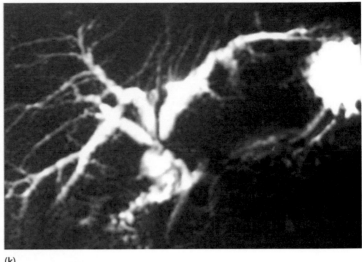

(j)   (k)

Figure 15.5 (Continued) **(j)** T-tube cholangiogram four weeks later shows a proximal duct narrowing. **(k)** MRCP performed three months after injury shows Bismuth Type IV stricture.

Summary of events

Common bile duct is misidentified as cystic duct because the fundus and the Hartman's pouch are not retracted in the recommended directions. This error lets the CBD to align with the infundibulum appearing as the cystic duct. Contrary to the standard guidelines, the dissection also takes place well below Rouviere's sulcus, thus making the bile duct vulnerable to injury. This misidentification further leads to dissection in the wrong plane i.e., medial to the bile duct. The duct and artery are divided without establishing the CVS, thus resulting in the division of the right hepatic artery and the CBD. The identification of CHD on subsequent dissection leads to the identification of the injury on the table.

Lessons learnt

- Adhering to basic principles of laparoscopic cholecystectomy, i.e., the proper retraction of the gallbladder, starting dissection above the plane of Rouviere's sulcus/the R4U line and dividing the structures ONLY after establishing the CVS could have possibly averted the injury.
- Right hepatic artery ligation and devascularisation of the common hepatic duct due to dissection leads to progression of low injury to a complex hilar injury.
- When vascular injury is suspected, definitive repair of the bile duct should be deferred till the ischemic injury manifests completely.

COMPLEX BILIOVASCULAR INJURY

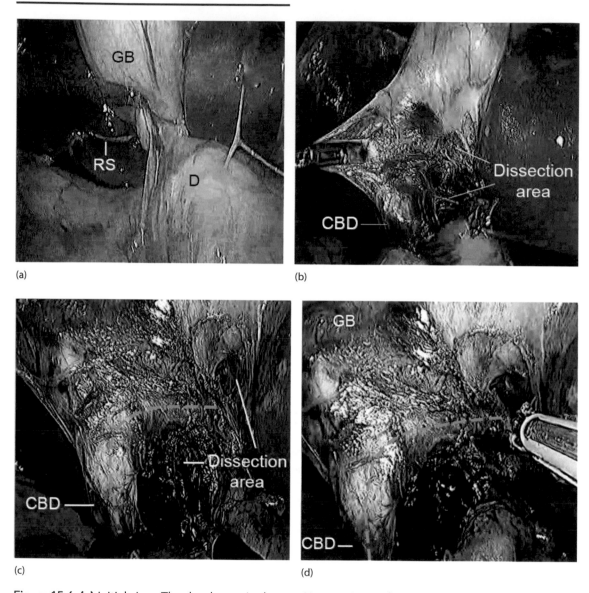

Figure 15.6 **(a)** Initial view. The duodenum is close to Hartman's pouch. Note Rouviere's sulcus. **(b)** Initial dissection is carried out medial to CBD up to the hilum. **(c)** The impression and course of the CBD/CHD (yellow dotted line) can be clearly made out. Extensive dissection has been performed with electrocautery medial to the common duct. **(d)** Near the hilum, the common hepatic duct (yellow dotted line) is mistaken as an artery and coagulated with bipolar forceps. *(Continued)*

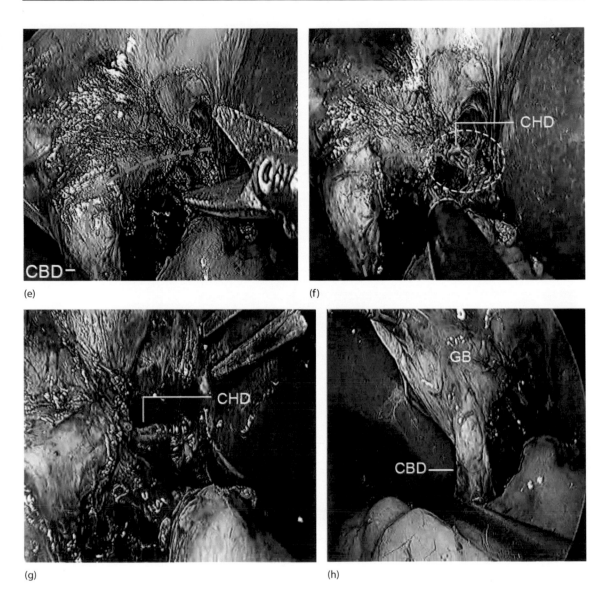

Figure 15.6 (Continued) **(e)** Coagulated structure is being divided with scissor. **(f)** Charred and transected common hepatic duct (dotted circle). **(g)** Significant bleeding is encountered as the dissection continues at the hilum. Control of bleeding is attempted with blind application of clips and monopolar coagulation. **(h)** The distal CBD, in continuity with the infundibulum, is mistaken as the cystic duct.   (Continued)

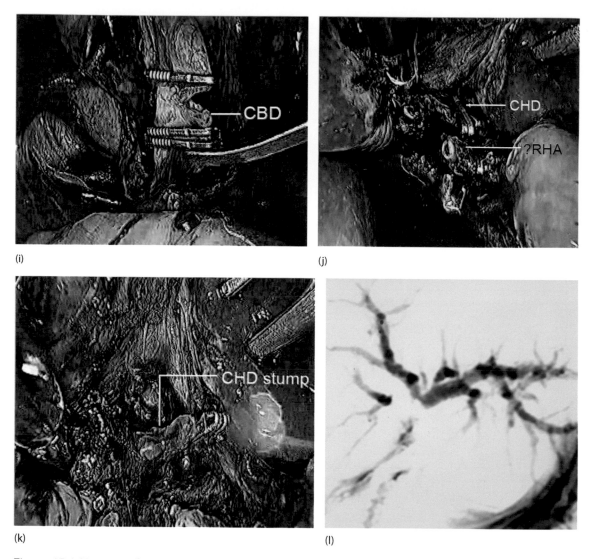

Figure 15.6 (Continued) **(i)** CBD is clipped and divided. **(j, k)** Hilar region after the transection of CHD and the vascular structures. Note the multiple clips on common hepatic duct stump and the right hepatic artery. **(l)** The resultant complex stricture (Bismuth Type V) on MRCP three months later. The transected duct at the hilum, separated right anterior, posterior and left hepatic ducts.

Summary of events

The common bile duct is misidentified as the cystic duct. Extensive dissection is carried out medial to CBD/CHD right up to the hilum. The common hepatic duct is misidentified as a blood vessel, coagulated with bipolar cautery and divided. On noticing the bile leak, clips are applied on the divided duct. To control bleeding during hilar dissection, blind clip application and cautery coagulation is carried out. The right hepatic artery is also coagulated, clipped and divided. Distally, the common bile duct is misidentified as the cystic duct because of its continuity with the infundibulum. It is clipped and divided. The "classic" complex bile duct injury with the excision of the long segment of the bile duct and vascular injury (HA) has resulted in this patient.

Lessons learnt

- Adhering to basic principles, i.e., proper retraction of the gallbladder, starting dissection above the plane of Rouviere's sulcus and dissecting close to the gallbladder to establish CVS can possibly avert the initial misidentification.
- Any wide tubular structure in the hepatocystic triangle should be viewed with the utmost suspicion and must be confirmed before subjecting to coagulation, clipping or division.
- Bile leak from the hilum warrants a strong suspicion of bile duct injury. Clip application without confirming the source of the leak should be avoided.
- Blind clip application and coagulation to control bleeding, specifically in the hilar area, must always be avoided.

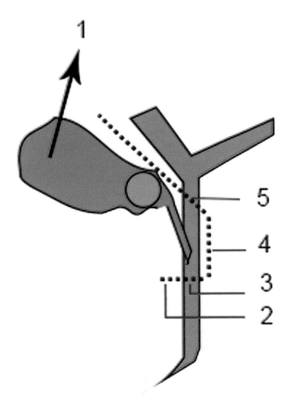

Figure 15.7 Schematic diagram explaining the most common mechanism and the sequence of events leading to bile duct injury. Dotted line represents the line of dissection. 1. Retraction of the gallbladder in the wrong direction (upwards and medially) narrows the hepatocystic triangle and brings the cystic duct into alignment with CBD, 2. Dissection starting at a lower plane (below the R4U line), 3. CBD, mistakenly identified as the cystic duct, clipped and divided, 4. Dissection proceeds medial to CBD, 5. Common hepatic duct is encountered, clipped and divided as dissection proceeds to the hepatocystic triangle to remove the gallbladder

Review of video and pictures and critical analysis of the events clearly leads us to draw the following conclusions. The key event is the "misidentification" of the CHD/CBD as the gallbladder or the cystic duct and dissection proceeding medial to the common duct, thereby endangering it.

The consistent "error" and subsequent injury can be avoided if the following steps are followed diligently during the cholecystectomy. These are the **Queen, King and Ace** of the prevention of bile duct injury.

Q. The precise direction of retraction of the fundus of the gallbladder (10 o'clock) and Hartmann's pouch (lateral and inferior) opens the hepatocystic triangle and retracts the gallbladder away from the CBD.

K. Identify the landmarks (Rouviere's sulcus and the cystic LN) and limit the dissection to the safe zone.

A. Do not divide ANY structure without demonstration of the 'Critical View of Safety'.

Summary and Recommendations

Cholecystectomy, although a low-risk procedure that can be offered as day care or short stay surgery, has the potential for serious complications. The large number of procedures performed across the world amplifies the burden of complications. Add to that the variable training and skills, the spectrum of pathologies and a wide variation of biliary anatomy increases the challenge in performing a safe cholecystectomy.

AUTHORS' RECOMMENDATIONS: TEN STEPS OF SAFE LAPAROSCOPIC CHOLECYSTECTOMY (*CHAPTER 3*)

1. High-definition camera, 30^0 telescope and a good camera operator.
2. Open pneumoperitoneum and port placement.
3. Traction of gallbladder
   a. 10 o'clock position (towards the right shoulder) of fundus
   b. Lateral and downward traction of Hartman's pouch.
4. Identify Rouviere's sulcus and other landmarks.
5. Open the posterior peritoneum to provide mobility to the gallbladder and to open the hepatocystic triangle.
6. Define safe area of dissection and achieve the CVS.
7. Time out
   a. Review the landmarks and anatomy
   b. Confirm the same with the team/senior colleague.

8. Clip and divide the cystic artery and the cystic duct.
9. Dissect gallbladder from the liver bed and place in a pouch.
10. Remove ports and close the fascial layer.

SOCIETY OF AMERICAN GASTROINTESTINAL & ENDOSCOPIC SURGEONS (SAGES) RECOMMENDATIONS

1. Use the 'Critical View of Safety' (CVS) method for the identification of the cystic duct and cystic artery during laparoscopic cholecystectomy.
2. Understand the potential for aberrant anatomy in all cases.
3. Make liberal use of cholangiography or other methods to image the biliary tree intraoperatively.
4. Consider an intraoperative momentary pause prior to clipping, cutting or transecting any ductal structures.
5. Recognize when the dissection is approaching a zone of significant risk and halt the dissection before entering the zone. Finish the operation by a safe method other than cholecystectomy if conditions around the gallbladder are too dangerous.
6. Get help from another surgeon when the dissection or conditions are difficult

THE MULTI-SOCIETY GUIDELINES FOR THE PRACTICE OF SAFE CHOLECYSTECTOMY[1]

Issues	Recommendations
1: Should the 'Critical View of Safety' (CVS) versus other techniques (e.g. infundibular, top-down, or intraoperative cholangiography) be used to mitigate the risk of bile duct injury (BDI) during laparoscopic cholecystectomy (LC)?	Surgeons should use the CVS for anatomic identification of the cystic duct and artery.
2: Should the fundus-first (top-down) technique versus subtotal cholecystectomy (STC) be used to mitigate the risk of bile duct injury when the CVS cannot be achieved during LC.	When CVS cannot be achieved and the biliary anatomy cannot be clearly defined by other methods (e.g., imaging) surgeons should consider STC over total cholecystectomy by the fundus-first (top-down) approach.
3: Should video documentation of the CVS (alone or in addition to operative notes) versus photo documentation (alone or in addition to operative notes) be used for limiting the risk or severity of BDI during LC?	No recommendation.
4: Should intraoperative biliary imaging versus no intraoperative biliary imaging be used for mitigating the risk of BDI during LC?	In patients with acute cholecystitis (AC) or a history of AC, liberal use of intraoperative cholangiography (IOC) during LC is recommended to mitigate the risk of BDI. Surgeons with appropriate experience and training may use laparoscopic ultrasound imaging as an alternative to IOC during LC. In patients with uncertainty of biliary anatomy or suspicion of BDI during LC, it is recommended that surgeons use intraoperative biliary imaging (in particular IOC) to mitigate the risk of BDI.
5A: Should intraoperative near-infrared (NIR) biliary imaging versus IOC be used for limiting the risk or severity of BDI during LC?	No recommendation
5B: Should intraoperative near-infrared biliary imaging with white light versus white light biliary imaging alone be used for limiting the risk or severity of BDI during LC	Near-infrared imaging may be considered as an adjunct to white light alone for identification of biliary anatomy during LC. However, relying on near-infrared imaging must not be a substitute for good dissection and identification technique

(Continued)

Issues	Recommendations
6: Should surgical (complexity) risk stratification v/s alternative or no risk stratification be used for mitigating the risk of BDI associated with LC?	A1: For patients with acute cholecystitis, surgeons may use the Tokyo Guidelines 18 (TG18), American Association of Surgery for Trauma (AAST) classification, or another effective risk stratification model for grading for severity of cholecystitis and for patient management. A2: During operative planning and intraoperative decision-making, surgeon should consider factors that potentially increase the difficulty of LC, such as male sex, increased age, chronic cholecystitis, obesity, liver cirrhosis, adhesions from previous abdominal surgery, emergency cholecystectomy, cystic duct stones, enlarged liver, cancer of gallbladder and/or biliary tract, anatomic variation, bilio-digestive fistula, and limited surgical experience.
7: Should risk stratification that accounts for cholecystolithiasis versus no/alternate risk stratification be used for mitigating the risk of BDI associated with LC?	No recommendation
8: Should immediate cholecystectomy defined as performed within 72 hours of symptom onset be used in acute cholecystitis (AC) versus delayed cholecystectomy? Delayed cholecystectomy is defined either as: (a) between 72 hours and 10 days after symptom onset; (b) 6–12 weeks after symptom onset; (c) greater than 12 weeks after symptom onset.	In patients presenting with mild AC, surgeon should perform LC within 72 hours of symptom onset. For patients with moderate and severe cholecystitis there is insufficient evidence to make a recommendation, particularly as it relates to the outcome of bile duct injury.
9: Should STC versus total laparoscopic or open cholecystectomy be used for mitigating the risk of BDI in marked acute inflammation or chronic biliary inflammatory fusion (BIF)?	When marked acute local inflammation or chronic cholecystitis with biliary inflammatory fusion (BIF) of tissues/tissue contraction is encountered during LC that prevent the safe identification of the cystic duct and artery, the surgeon should perform STC either laparoscopically or open depending on their skill set and comfort with the procedure
10: Should standard 4-port LC v/s reduced port LC (single incision LC, SILC) v/s robotic cholecystectomy v/s open cholecystectomy v/s other techniques be used for limiting the risk or severity of BDI in candidates for cholecystectomy?	For patients requiring cholecystectomy, use multi-port laparoscopic technique instead of single port/single incision technique.
11: Should interval LC versus no additional treatment be used for patients previously treated by cholecystostomy drainage?	In patients with AC previously treated by cholecystostomy who are good surgical candidates, interval cholecystectomy is preferred after the inflammation has subsided. For poor or borderline operative candidates, adopt non-surgical approach that may include percutaneous stone clearance through the tube tract or tube removal and observation if the cystic duct is patent.

(Continued)

Issues	Recommendations
12: Should conversion of LC to open cholecystectomy versus no conversion be used for limiting the risk or severity of BDI during difficult LC?	No recommendation.
13: Should surgeons take a time out to verify the CVS versus no time out be used for limiting the risk or severity of BDI during LC?	During LC, surgeon should take a momentary pause to confirm in his/her own mind that the criteria for the CVS have been attained before clipping or transecting ductal or arterial structures.
14: Should two surgeons versus one surgeon be used for limiting the risk or severity of BDI during LC?	No recommendation.
15: Should CVS coaching of surgeons versus no specific CVS coaching be used for limiting the risk or severity of BDI during LC?	Continued education of surgeons regarding the CVS during LC that may include coaching.
16: Should training of surgeons by simulation methods or video-based education versus alternative surgeon training be used for limiting the risk or severity of BDI during LC?	No recommendation.
17: Should more surgeon experience versus less surgeon experience be used for mitigating the risk BDI associated with LC?	To have a low threshold for calling for help from another surgeon when practical in difficult cases or when there is uncertain of anatomy.
18: For patients with bile duct injury during LC (in the OR or early postoperative period), should the patient be referred to a specialist with experience in biliary reconstruction or should the reconstruction be performed by the operating surgeon?	When BDI has occurred or is highly suspected at the time of LC or in the post-operative period, the surgeon should refer the patient promptly to another surgeon with experience in the management of BDI in an institution with a hepato-biliary disease multispecialty team. When not feasible to do so in a timely manner, prompt consultation with a surgeon experienced in the management of BDI should be considered.

THE SOCIETY OF ENDOSCOPIC AND LAPAROSCOPIC SURGEONS OF INDIA (SELSI)

The Society of Endoscopic and Laparoscopic Surgeons of India Guidelines (SELSI) has also come out with a set of guidelines for conduct of safe cholecystectomy that can be accessed in the corresponding document.[2,3]

NOTES

1 Brunt, L.M., Deziel, D.J., Telem, D.A. et al. Safe cholecystectomy multi-society practice guide-line and state of the art consensus conference on prevention of bile duct injury during chole-cystectomy. Annals of Surgery 2020; 272: 3–23.

2 Bansal, V.K., Misra, M., Agarwal, A.K. et al. SELSI consensus statement for safe cholecystectomy — prevention and management of bile duct injury — part A. Indian Journal of Surgery 2019. https://doi.org/10.1007/s12262-019-01993-2

3 Bansal, V.K., Misra, M., Agarwal, A.K. et al. SELSI consensus statement for safe cholecystectomy — prevention and management of bile duct injury — part B. Indian Journal of Surgery 2019. https://doi.org/10.1007/s12262-019-01994-1

Index

Page numbers in *italics* denote figures, those in **bold** denote tables